NIDRA YOGA FOR BEGINNERS

ELLA ROLANDO

LOWER STRESS, EASE PAIN, AND INCREASE PRODUCTIVITY WITH AWARE SLEEP

©2019

© 2019 Nidra Yoga for Beginners

All rights reserved. No part of the book may be reproduced in any shape or form without permission from the publisher.

This guide is written from a combination of experience and high-level research. Even though we have done our best to ensure this book is accurate and up to date, there are no guarantees to the accuracy or completeness of the contents herein.

ISBN: 9781703635874

Reviews

Reviews and feedback help improve this book and the author. If you enjoy this book, we would greatly appreciate it if you could take a few moments to share your opinion and post a review on Amazon.

Free Bonus
Yoga Nidra script

Go to **https://mailchi.mp/3b954c49187c/nidrayoga**, to download the guide for free

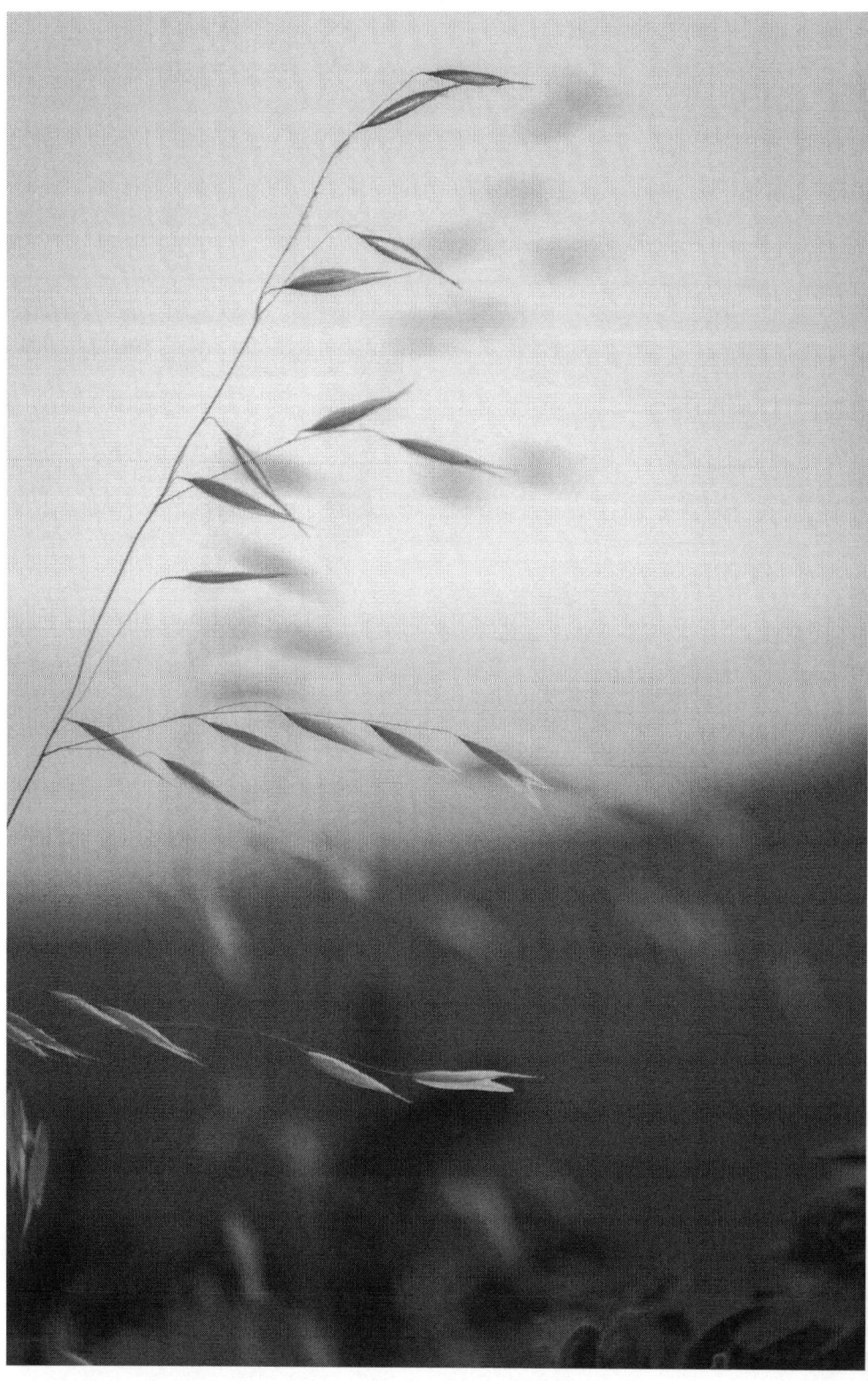

Table of Contents

Chapter 1: The Basics of Yoga Nidra   7
Chapter 2: History of Nidra   23
Chapter 3: Philosophy of Nidra   29
Chapter 4: Energetics & Essence of Nidra   35
Chapter 5: Benefits of Nidra   51
Chapter 6: Scripts of Nidra   67
Chapter 7: Build a Personal Practice   77
Chapter 8: 21-Day Challenge   101

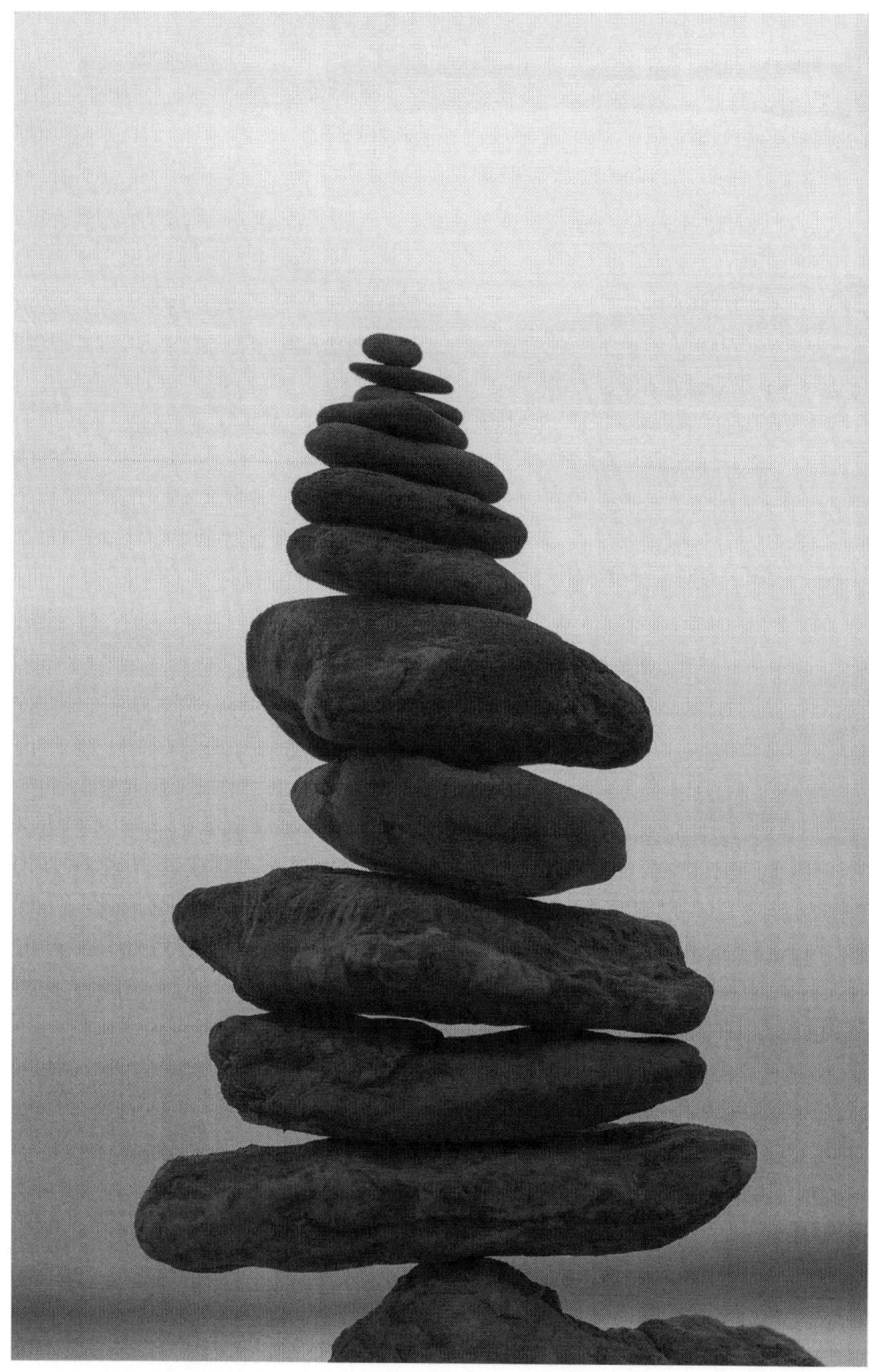

Chapter 1: The Basics of Yoga Nidra

"Yoga Nidra is the yoga of aware sleep. In this lies the secret of self-healing. Yoga Nidra is a pratyahara technique in which the distractions of the mind are contained and the mind is relaxed."

—Satyananda Saraswati

"Until you make the unconscious conscious, it will direct your life and you will call it fate."

—Carl Jung

Nidra Defined

What Nidra is:
- A somewhat meditative state, though it differs from many forms of meditation (more on that in a bit)
- A yoga practice with incredible benefits for *everyone*
- Something you can practice solo or in a yoga studio

What Nidra is not:
- A nap consisting of *deep* sleep (yes, the name "yogic sleep" is a bit misleading)
- An entirely traditional meditation
- Hypnosis

Yoga Nidra, or *yoganidrasana* in Sanskrit, translates to "Yogic Sleep Pose" or "Yogic Sleep." Nidra takes the practice of yoga outside of the physical asana shape, which typically looks similar to that of a Savasana posture. In a Yoga asana class—asana being the *physical* practice of yoga—you typically end in Savasana, a final meditation. The posture requires you to recline on your back with your legs extended and arms by your side. While you will likely recline down on your back in a similar manner to practice Nidra, the technique thrives as an entire practice in and of itself. You do not need to practice asanas, such as downward facing dog, prior to a Nidra session.

A Nidra practice induces yogis into a state of relaxation likened to that of natural sleep. The restful state brought about by even an hour-long practice of Nidra is thought to be equal to that of a full night's sleep, so it carries potent benefits within its methods. Nidra lovers return to the practice for numerous reasons, including the following:

- Combating insomnia
- Reducing stress
- Soothing anxious tendencies
- Enhancing awareness and a sense of "here, now"
- Instilling peace within one's mind and spirit
- A form of complementary medicine for the treatment of PTSD, depression, anxiety, and substance abuse

Sounds pretty desirable, right? Luckily, Nidra is not only beneficial in many ways, but it's growing in accessibility. If you've tried your hand at meditation in the past and perhaps did not love the rigidity of some methods, Nidra might be a more welcoming, flexible practice for you.

With Nidra, you can build your personal practice within the comfort of your own home and remain in a position that is comfortable for you throughout your journey. No need to sit up perfectly straight and stay in stillness despite aching to move; in fact, Nidra encourages comfort and will subtly shift your focus away from your physical body so that remaining in stillness is easier than ever.

A typical Nidra practice lasts anywhere from 30–45 minutes, and sometimes an entire hour or more. The student lies down on their back, and the teacher remains seated nearby as their guide. The teacher provides vocal cues to the student through the eight stages of the practice until their time together comes to a close.

Through the stages, the student's focus shifts and inner realms open within the student's reach. Inner realms relate to varying philosophical concepts, many of which will be explored in the pages to come. Nidra allows you to connect to your body beyond physical muscle, bone, and connective tissues. Exploring these energetic layers allows you to build a comprehensive yoga practice that can lead to enhanced overall well-being in mind, body, breath, and spirit.

Stages & Phases

Nidra contains a few specific phases which one shifts through over the course of usual practice. Studying each one in-depth can aid in your comfort and ability to actually move through each. Some of the characteristics of each phase may seem familiar, but in the past, you might not have been entirely conscious of the separation of each step, or its significance. Typically, teachers will not blatantly share which steps they are moving students through to minimize disruptions. But, when beginning to form a personal practice, awareness of the phases is a must.

Stage 1: Internalization

During this phase, the body shifts into a preliminary space for the preparation of moving into a Nidra state. This step allows you to set up *your* space as you would like. Place props where you would like them to rest in ways that will support your physical body as needed. While Nidra is often practiced while reclining, find a restful shape that works for you. Your Nidra shape might look entirely different from other yogis, and that is entirely okay. Release any last-minute physical wiggles before you settle into some semblance of stillness for a good while.

Stage 2: Sankalpa

Sankalpa translates to *affirmation*. Your Sankalpa is similar to an intention or mantra. Decide upon your Sankalpa quietly within your mind and being, based on how your energy feels today. Your affirmation should be chosen with care and intuition as your main guide, and you will focus on your Sankalpa throughout the practice. State your intention, within your mind, using the present or future tense. So, "I am" or "I will" might be the starting words of your

Sankalpa. Your Sankalpa remains with you and your practice until it becomes true and firmly grounded, realized in reality.

Stage 3: Rotation of Consciousness

Throughout this stage, notable shifts begin to occur. The concept of a "rotation of consciousness" simply means you will be shifting your focus from one body part to another, relaxing each part as you go. Your teacher will guide you with only their voice as they direct your inner gaze toward a specific body part. Typically, you begin on the right side of your body and progress to the left side. As you focus on each body part, the entirety of your breath and energy also shift toward it. Invite your body to settle in. You might tell your finger, thumb, hand, wrist, *relax, relax, relax*. Eventually, your entire body will reach a surrendered state. At first, this may be difficult, as we harbor far more tension in our physical bodies than we typically recognize. Let go of each body part, and feel the tension and stress flowing away from each part in succession.

Your sensory-motor cortex is activated during this phase as the rotation from part to part links to the *motor homunculus*. The *motor homunculus* is the little "being" or "voice" existing within your mind. Despite the shifting focus, you will remain physically still throughout stage three.

Stage 4: Breath Awareness

This stage might be more familiar if you have experience in other realms of yoga and meditation. As simple as it sounds, you will become more present and *in* your breath during stage four. Most of the time, during this stage your brain shifts from *beta* waves to *alpha* waves. The brain might also release endorphins that act as natural painkillers.

Stage 5: Manifestation of Opposites

While the first four stages are simple to understand in physical terms, stage five bears more complexities. The manifestation of opposites relates to the experience of simultaneous feelings or emotions arising within your body and mind. Emotional regulation and the sense of equanimity are stimulated during this experience. What brings about the awareness and sensations of opposition? The practice of *non-attachment* is responsible for such awakened perspectives. Through the cultivation of a consistent state of non-attachment, partly thanks to experiences such as Stage 5 in Nidra, you can deepen your yogic experience.

While moving through the exploration of oppositions, you might be guided into feeling incredibly heavy for a few moments —with cues telling you to "melt into your mat." A few beats later, after you feel as if you have all but sunk into the floorboards beneath you, you are told to *lighten, lighten, lighten*. You rise up and float away. With hardly a moment between the sinking and rising, you are experiencing opposites directly juxtaposed with one another.

Alternatively, you could experience the difference between fiery heat and tundra-cold. For a few moments, you are absolutely boiling hot, as if steeping in a cauldron. Before you know it, your bones are shivering and you might as well be standing in mile-high snowbanks.

Stage 6: Creative Visualization

Heading toward the end of a Nidra practice, stage six takes you into a space of guided visualization with a subtle creative flair sprinkled in by your teacher. You might be encouraged to explore the sensation of snowflakes cascading over the Rocky Mountains at one point. Moments later, you are seated on a beach with your toes kissed by the sea. Depending upon the teacher, this stage of the practice will vary.

Self-awareness develops and soothes any disturbing or intrusive thoughts or sensations. The thoughts which come to you naturally during this phase, from a peaceful realm, are known as the *samskaras* .

Stage 7: Sankalpa

Remember your earlier Sankalpa, the intention you set at the beginning of your practice? Now will be the time to draw it back to the forefront of your mind and reaffirm it within yourself. Allow it to permeate the depths of your being as you rest still within the realms of Nidra. At this point, your consciousness is more open than it was during stage two, so your Sankalpa can take root permanently.

Stage 8: Externalization

A fancy word, but really you will just be returning to a normal state of being. Grant yourself time, patience, and ease as you slowly wander out of the Nidra depths. Externalization can be incredibly jarring if you are not aware of your fragility. Honor your sensitive nature inherent to humanity. Let the light slowly find its way back into your visual perspective, and let your body find movement slowly and gently. Wiggle your fingertips, invite small movements into your physical space, and explore the purpose behind each intuitive pull to move.

Each of the eight stages holds its own space. When practiced with mindful cultivation and guidance, the stages begin to blend together into the whole of "Nidra." To further explore the stages and their elements and purpose within *your* practice, a 21-day guided journey can be found in Chapter 8.

The Purpose of Nidra

Nidra is a means of guiding a practitioner into a restful state between consciousness and deep sleep. Some folks compare the effects to that of lucid dreaming, so it might feel familiar to you. While practicing Nidra, your body seems to be asleep, but your consciousness rests in deepened awareness rather than unconscious rest. During typical nightly sleep cycles, your consciousness dials its awareness down from its typical waking thoughts. In Nidra, your awareness is increased within the energetic layers of your being beyond your thinking mind. Still, you are neither fully awake nor fully asleep.

By resting in this in-between state, your Parasympathetic Nervous System (PSNS) takes over, allowing for rest and digestion to occur. A parasympathetic state of "rest and digest" is necessary to balance the energy of the presently overactivated "fight-or-flight," or Sympathetic Nervous System (SNS). Our SNS tends to work in overdrive, thanks to the constant stimulation of our hustling Western cities. The PSNS has lost its effect as we find ourselves struggling to rest in such a state for the necessary amount of time for it to be of benefit. Nidra allows you the space and time for it to be profoundly beneficial, often more so than your usual night's sleep.

So, what exactly is the primary purpose of Nidra? Well, that is entirely up to you, the Yogi, since it is your path, after all. In its essence, Nidra aims to bring blissful rest and deepened awareness into your being through a simple practice accessible to all.

Nidra's Offerings

Minimization of Tension

We sit all day. We hold our hands in funky ways to carry our smartphones and tap, tap, tap away on our keyboards. Our physical habits, as 21st-century humans, are not conducive to fluidity and mobility.

Thankfully, through the stillness of Nidra, we can release tension through all our layers and shed away our growing rigidity. Resting in tension causes us to be more on-edge and in the zone of SNS, rather than the PSNS. Through the release of tension, our modern ways can come into balance. No need to toss your smartphone out the window (yet), as turning to Nidra might be the fix for you.

Tension tends to feed into stress, and vice versa. Stress then paves the way to other psychological and psychosomatic disorders. Both psychology and Eastern philosophy acknowledge three kinds of tension: muscular, emotional, and mental. All of these can be released in numerous ways, but Yoga Nidra alone can release all three in a single practice. Through breath awareness and rotation of consciousness, a yogi can melt into their mat and release their muscles. From there, emotions steady and smooth over. The mind quiets and the pacing of thoughts slows. Tension dissipates through the progressive relaxation methods inherently found in Nidra.

Another idea often heard in yoga communities is the idea that emotions, often those unprocessed or linked to trauma, remain in an individual's physical body until they are properly released. The hips are infamous for storing loads of tension related to emotions and experiences. Many students arrive at a variety of yogic practices with tight hips. It's sort of an unspoken state of being many people have come to accept. Mobile and fluid, though, is the way humans should move through the world. Our bodies are not meant to restrain us as much as they do when tension builds up in muscles and connective tissues.

As Nidra guides you further into your mind, you might witness emotions, experiences, and sensations long-buried or forgotten. Nidra asks you to confront these realms of yourself. Nidra nudges you further along so that you might release the tension and weight. These repressed memories, emotions, or energies can leave your physical body through the subtle practice of Nidra. Afterward, you might feel a bit vulnerable or exposed, but keep in mind, no one knows your inward journey but you. Unless you feel unsafe and need to talk to someone, you do not have to share your experience. The release of tension might be immediate for some, but a lot of the time it winds its way to you gradually. Be patient in the process of releasing deep-rooted tensions.

Stress levels, linked to general tension, have skyrocketed this century. Beyond our physicality, consider the state of our world: the powers that be—the connections (or lack thereof) we share between one another. We exist in a tension-filled state. With the news filling our screens, timelines, and televisions, we are more aware now than ever of tensions all around us.

With the idea of microcosmic shifts, related directly to your individual being, rippling outward to create macrocosmic effects, the release of tension through Nidra can move far beyond you. Your muscles, bones, and mind release, and the world might just be better for it. With that in mind, perhaps it's time to squeeze in some extra practice in hopes of achieving world peace?

Peace Within & Without

"Peace" is a sort of abstraction as it has a generalized connotation that disconnects a subjective perspective. We hear the word "peace" and immediately think of similar things—world peace, a peace sign made with one's fingers, the 1960s, hippies, etc. Through the exploration of the word and its direct meaning to you and you alone, you can come to experience it in a more intimate space while practicing Nidra.

One of the supposed benefits of Nidra is a cultivation of "inner peace," and this experience appears differently within every person. Sharing such sacred experiences can be difficult to put into words, so it makes sense that we rarely dig deeper into the true essence of peace.

Beyond the stereotypical images and feelings we, as a society, attribute to peace, what has your experience of peace been? What spaces, people, and rituals have brought you peace? What did peace look like for you? Was it energizing, soothing, or wildly blissful? While in Nidra, did you find peace at some point? Did it come about thanks to your acceptance of some hard truth or the release of an unprocessed experience? Through the careful introspection of singular words that we see all too often in the yoga world, you can further explore your personal journey.

After an experience of peace, how did you proceed? Did the peace remain within you, or did it dissipate shortly thereafter? Did you continue to seek a similar experience, or allow the next moment of "peace" to arrive naturally? No right or wrong answers exist for these questions. They are merely acting as guides for your moments of introspection.

Differentiating Nidra & the Many Meditation Styles

To get to the root of Nidra, let's begin by exploring the meditation techniques Nidra is *not*. Three popular methods of mindfulness meditation are Vedic Meditation, Vipassanā Meditation, and Loving-Kindness Meditation. Bear in mind, even yoga asana is often considered a meditation, but since that idea of an average vinyasa yoga class is not terribly difficult to differentiate from Nidra, we can leave that one out of this list.

Notable Qualities of Vedic Meditation, also known as *Transcendental Meditation*:

- Emphasis on the repetition of a mantra (a repeated word, affirmation, or phrase)
- Mantra is given to a student from a *guru*, or *spiritual guide*
- Student settles down with ease and can sit however they would like so long as their back is supported
- No strain to focus on anything in particular as the mantra naturally remains
- Eyes are closed
- When thoughts arise, you simply return to your mantra
- Typically practiced twice per day for approximately 20 minutes each session

Notable Qualities of Vipassanā Meditation:

- Emphasis on exploring inner energetic layers and yet-to-be-discovered aspects of self
- Practiced while seated with a tall spine, slightly engaged core muscles, and legs crossed
- Careful attention paid to physical sensations, breath is "sent" or "directed" toward any physical sensation until it eventually lessens
- Observation remains steady on physical sensation and breath throughout
- Practice for an extended period of time, often in a retreat setting where Noble Silence (non-speaking, non-engaging) is practiced at the same time
- Eyes are closed

Notable Qualities of Loving-Kindness Meditation:

- Emphasis on feelings of warmth, goodness, and compassion
- Focus on sending love and compassion toward others, rather than focusing on self alone
- Exploration of the inner experience of love and kindness
- A Buddhist technique
- Practiced for a few minutes at least once per day
- Eyes are closed
- Relatively relaxing
- Repetition of a positive phrase

Notable Qualities of Yoga Nidra:

- A progressive technique aiming for deep relaxation which will lead to greater awareness following a practice
- Repetition of a mantra, but only at certain points (two phases, to be exact)
- Some focus on the physical body, but only during one phase
- Some exploration of the mind, but only during one phase
- Often practiced while reclining down on your back
- Eyes are closed
- Props can be used to support your body

- Typically practiced for 30–60 minutes, 45 minutes on average

Nidra is not your usual meditation. You could sit with perfect posture and regulate your breath and perhaps find yourself experiencing similar side effects to that of Nidra, but that's not wholly Nidra. Nidra allows you to rest comfortably in your space and you typically recline on your back. Your breath will be your focus for a bit, but will not remain as such for the entire session.

After some breath awareness, you are guided into the proper state by a teacher. This "proper state" is one in between "awake" and "asleep." You will repeat a mantra a few times over to ingrain it in your mind before moving ahead. The practice then shifts depending upon the teacher. In some cases, you might hear your teacher's voice for the entire session. They might guide you through specific guided visualizations that will encourage you to explore your mind, breath, and energetic body as they cue. Other teachers might grant you ample space to rest in silence. While resting in a silent, Nidra state, you would be entrusted to guide yourself. It might take a good amount of consistent practice to arrive at a space where you feel comfortable taking such control over your practice.

With a teacher's guidance and through the cultivation of your practice, you become increasingly aware of your body and allow it to relax entirely. In doing so, while keeping your "mind's eye" or "inner focus" on your breath, you can come to rest in the deeper level of awareness, which remains the goal throughout the entire practice. You might stop focusing on your breath and your physical body when practicing Nidra as intended.

In this way, Nidra does mimic sleep, as you are unaware of your body and are not actively regulating your breath. All bodily functions continue automatically, without your control. Your teacher remains present with you throughout your Nidra practice, but you will very rarely be aware of their direct presence.

Nidra differs from the Savasana of which you might be familiar. Occurring at the end of a Yoga asana practice, Savasana, or "Corpse Pose" acts as a final meditation and relaxation period. Nidra typically occurs as a "class" entirely on its own. Despite the similar body position —reclined on your back —the two are not the same. Nidra is not a "super long Savasana." Rather, Nidra allows for awareness to reach and sustain a level of relaxation that typically would not occur during the majority of Savasana experiences. At its core, Savasana is an asana, yogic posture itself. In most philosophies, Nidra is the entire practice itself and not only an asana shape you create on your mat.

Further, the practice of Nidra exists in a different realm than the well-known Dream Yoga method within Tibetan Buddhism. Dream Yoga, also known as Milam, is the Yoga of the Dream State and a form of tantric Sadhana. Sadhana means "daily spiritual practice." While Nidra might be a part of your Sadhana, it is not synonymous with Dream Yoga and the tantric path. The work of ancient scholars and philosophers throughout different regions within Eastern countries allowed for similar practices to be cultivated with a nearly identical "end point." This endpoint tends to liken itself to enlightenment —the state of pure bliss and alignment with a God or Spirit energy. While the paths leading to enlightenment are similar, the methods and techniques are practiced differently.

Drawing similarities between Nidra and Dream Yoga is hardly far-fetched, as the link between dreamtime and the "sleep" aspect of Nidra is quite visible. At its roots, Dream Yoga stems from Tibetan monks and follows a direct line from teacher to student. Nidra is a bit more broad, as it has spread more widely, and its roots mainly stem from Hinduism, though some links to Buddhism can be seen.

Nidra's Presence in Western Society

The quote shared by Carl Jung, renowned psychoanalyst, at the beginning of this book demonstrates a philosophy shared by many people: "Until you make the unconscious conscious, it will direct your life, and you will call it fate." Some yogis interpret this to mean that Jung is hinting at the imbalances seen in our world and our inability to face such realities. Instead of gazing inward and facing a rather harsh truth about the state of the world, and ourselves in some ways, we choose to allow burdens and imbalances to carry us forward. Rather than admitting that what guides us is important and worth looking into, we claim it to be "fate." Fate is notoriously impossible to meddle with, so why fight it? Jung makes the case that the work is worthwhile, for in facing the unconscious depths you can gain remarkable control over your path.

With the Western world heading toward automation and its masculine-based Yang-tendencies— fast-paced and relentless, holding steady into the decades to come, many folks find themselves craving an awakening of sorts. For many, these cravings are satisfied by the practice of Eastern philosophy, medicine, and spirituality. With an emphasis on Yin, the feminine energy which dances with masculine "Yang," Eastern values have experienced a Renaissance in the Western world. In recent decades, Buddhism, Hinduism, Daoism, Yoga asana, meditation, and Eastern medicine have meandered into mainstream culture and discourse.

The concepts of "masculine" and "feminine" energy exist beyond the ideas of gender, sexuality, and identity when placed in the context of spirituality. Mainly, they are used to categorize a variety of energetic sensations and experiences. A person who identifies as a man might relate to a fair amount of feminine qualities, while a woman might relate to more masculine qualities. The energetics are always shifting and *can* be shifted through yogic practices such as Nidra. If someone who felt more masculine practiced Nidra, they might feel more "feminine" and "Yin" after the practice due to Nidra being inherently feminine.

For clarity, Yin, the feminine, and Yang, the masculine, can be compartmentalized as follows:

Yin

Feminine

Lunar

Cool

Still

Dark

Night

Slow

Moon

Intuitive

<u>Yang</u>

Masculine

Solar

Warm

Active

Light

Day

Fast

Sun

Logical

When thinking about the energetics of Yin and Yang, keep the Yin and Yang symbol in mind. The two cannot exist without one another. Consider the duality of Yin and Yang, rather than seeing them as polar opposites. Within the swirl of black Yin, a white dot of Yang floats. And, within the swirl of white Yang, a black dot of Yin holds steady. Within the Yang there is Yin, and within the Yin there is Yang. Neither is "good" nor "bad," they simply are a means of allowing greater insight to a yogi's state of balance or imbalance. The aim is to come into a state of balance when dealing with Yin and Yang.

If you notice you are incredibly overworked, spending long hours on your computer, and feeling as if your nerves are fried, you might be embracing too much Yang. To find balance, you can invite some Yin practices into your days. You might not start by meditating for hours on end, as that would then be *too much* Yin, but a few minutes per day might allow the Yin within the Yang to grow. When Yang maintains dominance for too long, burnout becomes all too common. Take a moment and consider the present state of the Western world. Despite the Eastern concepts woven in, would you agree we live in a Yang-dominant society?

Still, despite what might be considered overly Yang, yogic concepts seem to be grounded in their present popularity. While trends in the practice of physical yoga shift year to year (one year, Hot Yoga, the next, Vinyasa Flow, and then, Hatha), new practices continue to flourish under the radar. These include Yin Yoga, founded by Paul Grilley, and Yoga Nidra, founded by Swami Satyananda. With their offerings of bliss, deep restoration, and a slower pace, they now fill the schedules of studios across the States alongside the fast-paced, Vinyasa Flow–inspired classes.

The conscious world, littered with masculine-tendency and an accepted love for such masculinity, craves the energetically feminine ways of Yin and Nidra in an unconscious manner that has risen to the forefront of our minds in recent years. Until we make such unconscious yearning for a slower ritual, a more fulfilling daily life, and deepened awareness, society might continue to unfurl down a destructive path. The growing popularity of the slowing qualities of Nidra is a means of society's members expressing their need for healing more unconsciously. Nonetheless, this shift toward Nidra has allowed for the practice to spread widely and drip into more people's lives. With the numerous benefits of Nidra only growing, there is no limit to the relief one may feel from this practice.

Pause for a moment. Envision a world where the majority of folks allow for the time to partake in (or even simply share the concept of) the practice of Nidra each day. Our modern daily lives would likely be a lot more grounded and abundant in the experience of peace and relaxation. Envision a world where the majority of folks are actively considering their emotions, state of mind, and finding ways to remain balanced. Without stress and anxiety running rampant, where would our world be?

A rise in Nidra is a return to the roots which offer healing, bliss, and well-being for all. Thus, the recent surge in popularity is of benefit to everyone, and in curating your Nidra practice, you can be part of an effort to heal our modern Western world. Thanks to Nidra, you can lower your stress levels, deepen your sleep, stimulate your creativity, and find yourself a bit more awake and aware on a day-to-day basis. Make the unconscious, conscious and watch the Earth, and your deadline-chasing ways, shift magically.

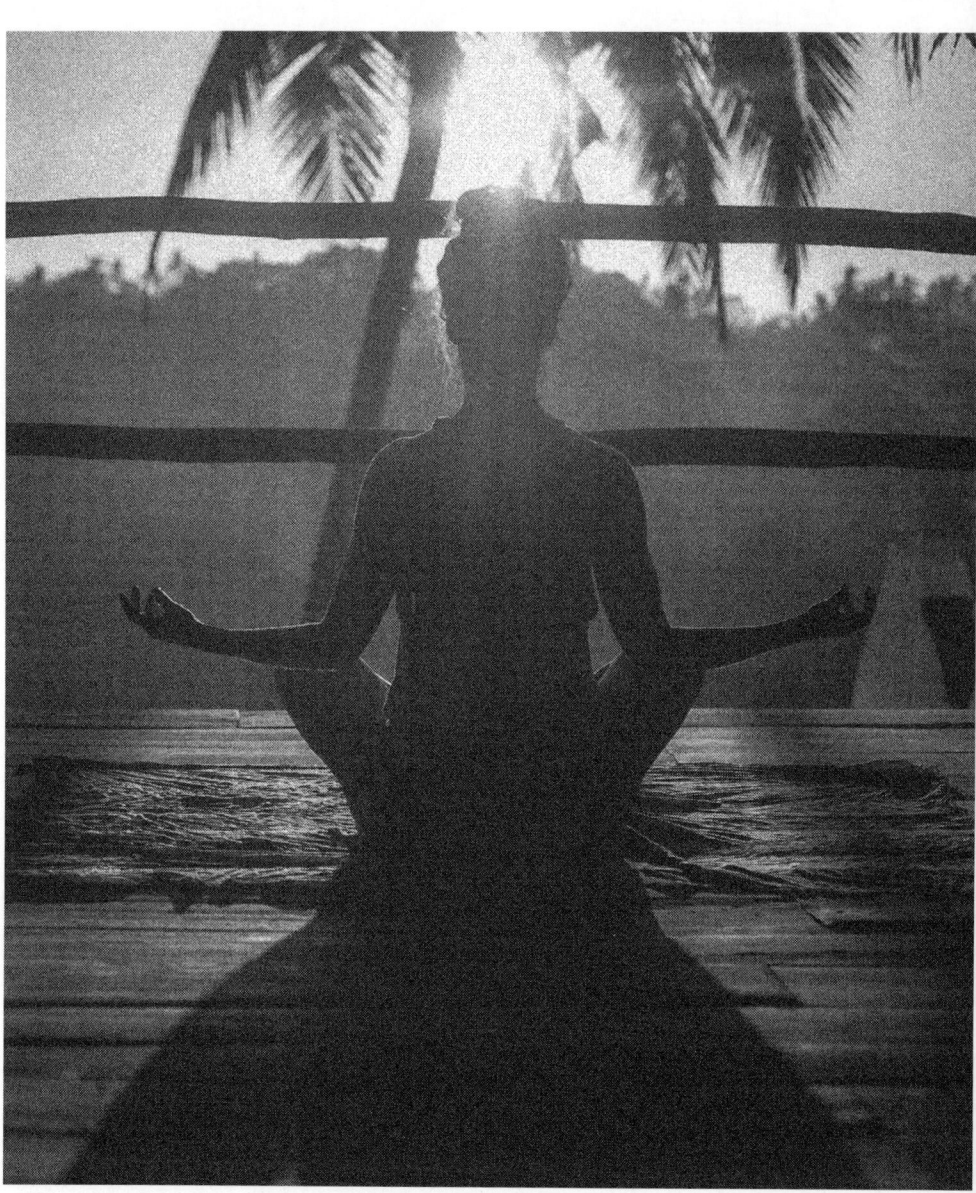

Chapter 2: History of Nidra

Eastern Roots

As in most Yogic practices, Nidra came into being in the Eastern regions of our world. Swami Satyananda Saraswati brought modern Nidra into its present form while spending his days at a Vedic school in Rishikesh, India. With Rishikesh considered the Yoga capital of the world, this comes as little surprise. Ancient texts, teachers, and wisdom fill the lands and minds of Rishikesh.

Dial the clock back a fair bit further back, though, and references to Nidra were there, tucked away in ancient tantric texts. Tantra, meaning "weave," exists beyond just the literal meaning many have come to use as its sole definition. Woven into its modern incarnation by both Hinduism and Buddhism, tantra is an esoteric, "mysterious" tradition. The tantric path is complex and mystifies many. With Vishnu, Shiva, and Shakti as some of tantra's main pillar, and an emphasis on mantra, meditation, yoga, and ritual; tantra came about from numerous paths and can be practiced in many different manners. Thus, the word "tantra" meaning "weave" makes sense. Weaving together many concepts and philosophies, tantra is a freeing and often enlightening path which utilizes ancient rituals drawn from scholarly tantric texts to lead a practitioner through their Sādhanā. Sādhanā is your daily yogic practice. Sometimes it could appear as a day of reading books such as this, and another day it might be a physical yoga practice.

Many practices used by modern yogis came about from Tantra. Mudras, for one, came about from the tantra texts. Mudras are physical gestures most often made with the fingers and hands. They are meant to lock in a specific essence in the physical body while facilitating energy flow within the subtle body. Mudras can aid in a yogi's exploration through their inner realms. Nidra finds itself rooted in tantra alongside some vividly beautiful company.

The story of how Swami became aware of the mental state reached in Nidra is fascinating. While at the Vedic school in Rishikesh, Swami Satyananda would guard the school at times.

This duty required Swami to remain awake throughout the night. Eventually, he would succumb to sleep around 3 a.m. and stay in such a restful state until about 6 a.m. The boys attending the Vedic school would wake up at 4 a.m. to chant Sanskrit prayers, or "mantras." One would assume Swami might not be aware of such chanting; he was, after all, fast asleep after having stayed up rather late into the night. Surprisingly, Swami was still able to absorb most of the mantras chanted by the young students, even while sleeping. Such remembrance took him by surprise, as he had never read those exact mantras, but still, they had found their way permanently into his mind.

Swami approached the guru of the school and shared this strange occurrence with him. The guru was not as surprised as Swami. While asleep, he told Swami, you were able to register the mantras within your subtle body, or "emotional body," thanks to the repetition of the mantras by the boys. Now, you might be thinking, "Does that mean I can take a nap and absorb all the information in this book?" Perhaps you could, but Swami had not yet found his way to Nidra's truth just yet.

With the guidance of the guru, Swami took to the ancient texts lining the shelves of the Vedic school. Most of these texts had tantric roots and would lead him down the path toward Nidra. The exact dates aligning with Swami's realization and Nidra studies are unknown, but appear to have occurred sometime in the mid-twentieth century.

Due to recent revelations, Swami Satyananda Saraswati's actions cannot remain unmentioned in full disclosure alongside his writings and teachings. Sexual abuse allegations were presented to the global yoga community in 2014 and some called for a boycott of Swami's literature.

Ancient Texts

The earliest textual reference to Nidra seems to have been written down in or around 700 BC. Of course, before humans took pen to paper and jotted down their thoughts and visions for their world, oral traditions were the primary source of carrying and sharing knowledge. So, Nidra likely originated around 1,000 BC, with the essence of the practice passed down through oral storytelling.

Despite being brought to the modern world by Swami Satyananda, Nidra is far older than he. Still, we owe great thanks to Swami for his work in curating modern Nidra and allowing it to find its way into our Western culture.

Lineage

Ancient practices came about simultaneously, in most cases. No singular person can be credited with the creation of Yoga Nidra, but the big names in the game are worthy of receiving an acknowledgment. As mentioned beforehand, Swami Satyananda is responsible for the resurgence of Nidra in recent decades. Swami once wrote, "the present system of Yoga Nidra, which I have devised, enables people who are unfamiliar with Sanskrit mantras to gain the full benefits of the traditional Nyasa. It can be beneficially practiced by people of any religion or culture."

For reference, "Nyasa" means an awakening of subtle energy. When Swami experienced the mantras entering his consciousness through his subtle body, Nyasa was occurring without him realizing.

When discussing Nidra with some teachers, many will not acknowledge Swami as the founder. While this is entirely valid in many ways, as the practice stretches back centuries before Swami came to find it, his work remains pertinent to the modern ways in which Nidra benefits us all.

Some twenty-first-century scholars have gone so far to doubt Swami's Nidra origin story. Dr. Mark Singleton expressed his doubts vividly and claims that Swami exaggerated the tantra roots he tied to Nidra. Rather, Dr. Singleton believes much of the practice can be linked to twentieth-century therapies, primarily Western relaxation methods. While it is immensely vital to honor the Eastern cultures from where these Western methods came about, Singleton's claims may be valid. Throughout the mid-twentieth century, Western culture and Eastern philosophy were beginning to mingle and meld around the world. Eastern practices had begun to fall under the influence of Western ideals. Swami's guru at the Vedic school taught a Western relaxation practice created by Edmund Jacobson. Jacobson's method taught a progressive relaxation technique. Some semblance of similarity to Nidra is not too difficult to see.

Plus, the concept of "relaxation" was not entirely born of the Eastern world, as Westernized yoga brought relaxation into the picture. Before yoga wound its way to the West, the emphasis was placed upon varying "end goals," but blissful relaxation was never in the mix. As much of modern tantra is a melting pot of thoughts and rituals from different regions, perhaps it's entirely fair to say the same of Nidra.

In more recent years, Dr. Richard Miller, a clinical psychologist, developed an even more modernized means of practicing Nidra. Dr. Miller created iRest (Integrative Rest), a system used primarily as a therapeutic practice. iRest greatly benefits the likes of hospital patients, prisoners, and war veterans.

Integrative Rest, otherwise known as "iRest," offers mindfulness meditation geared toward specific communities and populations. In 2011, L. Stankovic, whose research is based at John F. Kennedy University, conducted an eight-week study. In this study, researchers examined the possibilities and efficacy of offering weekly iRest classes to local military veterans at a nearby San Francisco Bay Area community mental health agency. With ages ranging from forty-one to sixty-six, the implementation of iRest was a success. Eleven participants completed the study in full and reported reduced rage, anxiety, and emotional reactivity. Plus, they felt more at peace, aware, and relaxed even when experiencing intrusive memories and other symptoms related to PTSD. All of the eleven participants shared that they would continue to attend iRest classes once per week if it were available to them.

With PTSD running rampant through our society, mainly in military combat veterans and those recovering from sexual trauma and general abuse, curating healing methods is a must. iRest can be made easily accessible to communities seeking such shifts in mental state and overall being. With Nidra offered to populations that might have previously felt shunned from other Yoga practices, for a variety of reasons, more individuals can find healing through Eastern practices.

As noted earlier, Nidra offers psychosomatic healing, which connects the body and the mind in their healing. Despite the physical stillness in Nidra, you are still able to find healing through gentle awareness of your physical body. Somatic psychology builds upon the idea that our bodies can heal us. Through a holistic approach, somatic psychotherapy offers a philosophy similar to that of Nidra—it eases you into physical sensation and then moves into subtle energy layers. In somatic psychotherapy, an individual might practice dance therapy, EMDR (eye movement desensitization processing), or yoga asana in order to move stagnant energy within themselves. The stagnant energy might show up as tightness in hips, but it really relates to blockages in the subtle, energetic body that cannot be "felt" in the same way as the physical muscle and joints.

EMDR's elements are rather similar to the visualization of Yoga Nidra, as they ask a practitioner to focus their mind in a certain way to enhance a sensation or arrive in a specific state of mind. Whereas EMDR focuses directly on a past trauma or experience, Nidra asks you to rest with your Sankalpa, a chosen mantra, in mind and allow it to hold your focus. By learning these methods, a student can unlearn past narratives and restructure their perspective.

Nidra has come a long way from being stifled and stuck in the pages of ancient texts tucked upon shelves, left to gather dust. Whether you're new to the Yogic world or not, perhaps you can tap into the beauty that is the consistent progression of ancient wisdom into modern-day contexts. By allowing older methods such as Nidra to flourish, we are building a connection to wells of ancient healing and joy that have been left untapped for far too long. The murky depths of Nidra are vast, and Nidra welcomes with an open spirit anyone who wishes to explore.

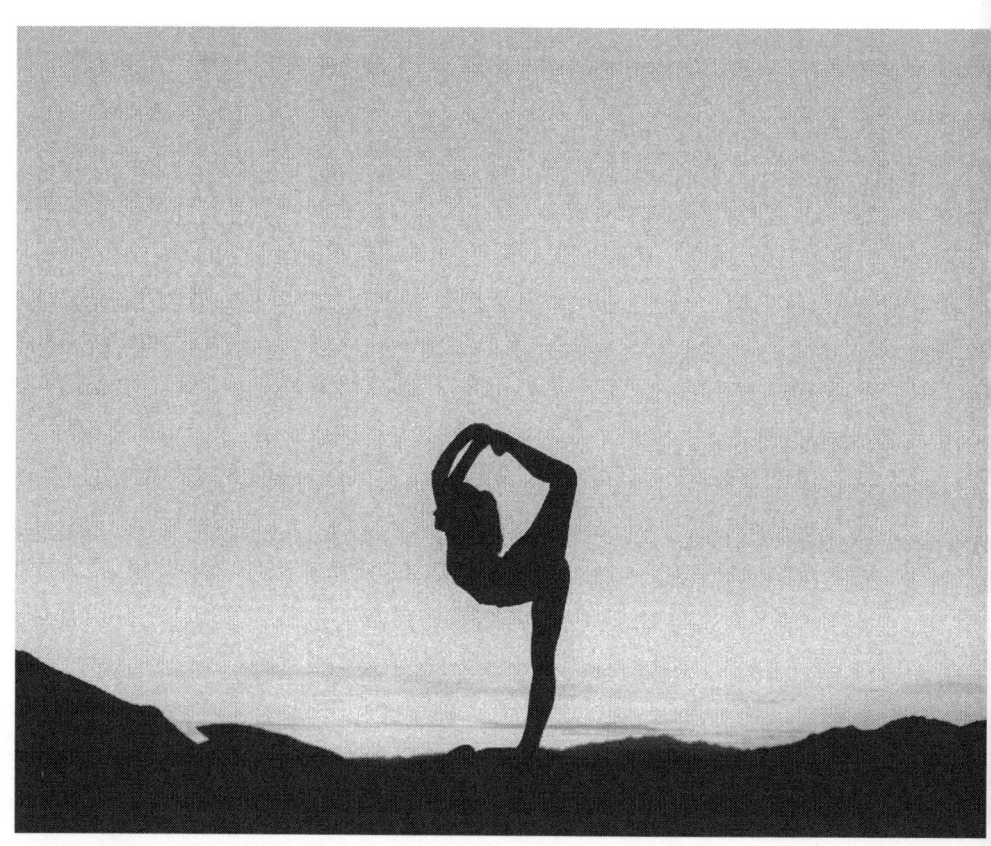

Chapter 3: Philosophy of Nidra

"At the point of sleep when sleep has not yet come, and external wakefulness vanishes, at this point being is revealed."—Vijñāna Bhairava Tantra, ancient tantra text

Indian Concept

Within the realms of Nidra, there are two subgroups. The first falls purely under Indian belief systems and practices. Texts dating back to the Middle Ages detail methods similar to that of modern Yoga Nidra. Despite the dated pages, the information remains accessible and beneficial to this day.

Some of these Indian texts rely entirely on philosophical thought, while others are a bit more mythologically based. Either way, both routes agree that Nidra is linked to Vishnu, an Indian God. Vishnu, one of the principal Hindu deities, represents absolute truth. He preserves the energy of the universe. In one tale from Hindu mythology, Vishnu sleeps at the moment when creation, or "life," is destroyed. While Vishnu sleeps, he experiences the moment in between life and destruction. It's thought that Vishnu guides the universe, so when he rests, the universe's life force shrinks into a new form. It's in this space that a state of being occurs similar to that of Nidra—both are between full life and rest.

Modern interpretations of Nidra differ slightly, but the sleeping concept lingers in the present discourse and in Swami Satyananda's discovery of the practice. When a Nidra yogi rests in between sleep and usual consciousness, they are the universe resting a bit. Such is believable if you tap into the idea that human beings, and all life, are born of the universe and play out their days as the universe in motion. Human minds come into Nidra and are able to consume, as Vishnu would, some amount of Divine, universe-born energy. In doing so, a higher state of consciousness is achieved. This heightened state might be felt or experienced in varying ways depending on the given yogi.

Tantra Technique

The second subsection of Nidra's roots takes us back to tantra. To reiterate, tantra is a path built for uplifting consciousness and connecting to higher energetics of being. The goal of Nidra is entirely up to the yogi practicing the method, but within the context of tantra, the purpose is detailed and targeted with greater precision by the practitioner.

Whereas a general Yoga practice—consisting of the occasional breathwork practice, a brief daily meditation, and a proper amount of asana—might eventually bring a yogi to a blissful state, tantra subtly guides you further within. Tantric methods encourage yogis to practice deeply diving into the inner realms and their own energetic landscapes to raise their understanding of self. Following such explorations, through meditation, Nidra, or ecstatic movement, the self rises to a higher state of consciousness. Eventually, through sequential experiences of such expansion and transcendence, one might liberate themselves.

The majority of tantra experiences are unique to an individual, therefore much of the practice remains shrouded in an alluring mystery. Perhaps, this is why the sexual aspects of the path have grown to be how tantra is widely known. With the knowledge that tantra is deeply personal and inclusive of a wide array of practices, one begins to understand how deep the methods run.

While walking the tantra path, teachers guide you along the way, as they likely would on any spiritual path. Their grip, though, is subjectively loosened in comparison to other routes and means of spiritual enlightenment and liberation. Tantric yogis hold a steady understanding of the ebb and flow of the spiritual path upon which they have embarked. There exists an appreciation of impermanence, the give and take of all energy, and how teachers, students, and peers will come and go. With that in mind, tantra's links to modern Nidra become more apparent.

As mentioned earlier on, Nidra differs from most other meditations due to the teacher's detachment and distant guidance compared to that of a more rigid and "traditional" meditation practice. With such distance, students are welcomed into their inner realms by themselves and left to their own means to explore the walls and halls within themselves. Teachers remain present, but the grip remains loose, as is the case with much of the tantra path.

A tantra teacher of mine once shared, "You can only take others as far as you have gone." Whether you are teaching, sharing, or practicing purely for your benefit, such wisdom rings true. Tantra and Nidra practices both invite practitioners to wander their personal depths and darkness. Such a trip within is no easy task and requires a steady mind. Thankfully, the relaxation aspects of Nidra allow for the darkest depths of self to be revealed slowly. A gentle unfurling comes about while practicing Nidra, and other tantra rituals play out similarly.

Within the context of tantra, Yoga Nidra allows you to find ease in stillness and invites you to wander the depths of your mind and Spirit softly. All the while, you walk a path toward higher consciousness and deepen your connection to the Divine, or "Spirit" energy.

Modern Development

Contemporary Nidra continues to find itself wound into the Western world, similar to most other Yogic practices. When practicing Yoga Nidra, educating yourself on the history of the method remains an immensely important aspect of the practice, perhaps equal to that of the Nidra itself. As a Westerner benefiting from this Eastern practice, pausing to acknowledge the cultural roots and history is worthwhile.

While embarking on the path of curating your Nidra practice, weaving in ancient wisdom will only be beneficial, never detrimental. Knowing the depths of the practice and being able to discuss it with vigor and from a space of well-versed education will add respect, diligence, and integrity to your entire Yoga practice. Despite Nidra being reasonably new to the Western world, it did come about when Eastern practices had already begun to be washed over in Western languages and customs. At first, it might be a bit difficult to pick apart the authentic aspects from the inauthentic. It's the attempt to honor the practice with a genuine and respectful approach that will make all the difference.

As you curate your Nidra practice, seek out authentic resources, such as the teachers and the ancient texts mentioned beforehand. Dig deep into your Sadhana beyond the meditative and physical methods. After all, Nidra came about thanks to some ancient Indian scholars digging deep into their minds and then sharing it onto paper in the hopes that their written words might inspire future generations to peruse the literature. Study these texts, as the ancient scholars wished for you, and be sure to explore within—and beyond—the self and watch your life expand beyond what you once knew to be possible and true.

Technological Insight

Thanks to modern technological advancements, Nidra's effects on the brain can be seen with greater clarity and validity. Not only does the practice create a feeling of balance in your nervous system, but technology allows us to see why such shifts happen. You're able to understand conceptually, and actually see the changes in your brain waves, with the correct technology.

Through the conscious arrival into a restful state, your brain waves slow. Your brain waves move from a beta state, awake and lively, to an alpha state, relaxed and present. Alpha waves are the more restorative "setting" for your brain and allow for the blissful rest of Nidra to saturate your entire being. Alpha waves are linked to dream states and REM sleep, so you're floating about within that space. Higher theta waves occur at this level too and have been linked to advanced and more rewarding learning abilities, such as those experienced when Swami Satyananda was able to learn the mantras as easily as he did in his state of sleep. He had the relaxation-induced theta waves to thank for his receptivity.

The realm where theta waves dance is one where a sort of void exists. If you've ever been asleep and heard the voices of someone in an adjacent room, and their presence melded into your dreams in some way, *that* was likely due to the imaginative ways of theta waves. The in-between state of wake and deep sleep brings you into one of the brain's most creative states. "Nothing" is not occurring yet, but "everything" is not occurring either. Take a minute to process that, read the sentence again maybe. It's a funny concept to grasp at first, that's for sure. Think of it this way: when you are floating on your back in the ocean, part of you remains receptive to the sunlight on the front of your body. The other "half" of you connects deeply to the inner realms—the deep, dark parts of the ocean that exist underwater. Part of you exists in between the two, with an awareness of both the sun and the water at once. Nidra exists in a similar in between, where you are able to receive both sensations somewhat equally and experience the *melding* of the two together.

Following the theta waves, delta waves arrive. Delta waves offer the most restful state of being. Thanks to their peaceful energy, the "rest and digest" state properly begins and lets your organs rest a bit, your stress hormones slow, and your overall physical body succumbs to deep sleep.

Beyond delta waves, Nidra shows you waves that are typically inaccessible during your normal sleeping pattern. This fourth state expands beyond the nothingness of theta waves and transcends the rest of delta waves. The state exists as one of heightened consciousness where you are far and away from tangible reality and any awareness of your physical body. Such a state might sound daunting or frightening, especially upon first hearing of its existence. With diligent practice and the cultivation of your Nidra practice, though, it comes with ease and is comforting, rather than alarming.

One crucial piece of advice for any aspiring yogi is to take your time in cultivating your practice. Not every practice will feel the same as any other. A main key to carry with you throughout your exploration of Nidra's many blessings is that of *equanimity*. Equanimity means "mental calmness" or "composure." When put in the context of a meditation technique or Yogic practice, Nidra included, it acts as a framework of mind for each and every practice.

As you traverse your inner realms, accept all you witness without reaction or judgment. Avoid labeling experiences as "good" or "bad." If you have a particularly enlightening practice one day, seeking something exactly like it again will only hold you back. Approach each moment of your practice without expectation. Allow for the fluidity, the Yin aspects of Nidra, to flood your practice so that it has the space to unfurl as it wishes. Nidra acts as a guide in many ways, so trust the ancient wisdom, go forward, and wander within.

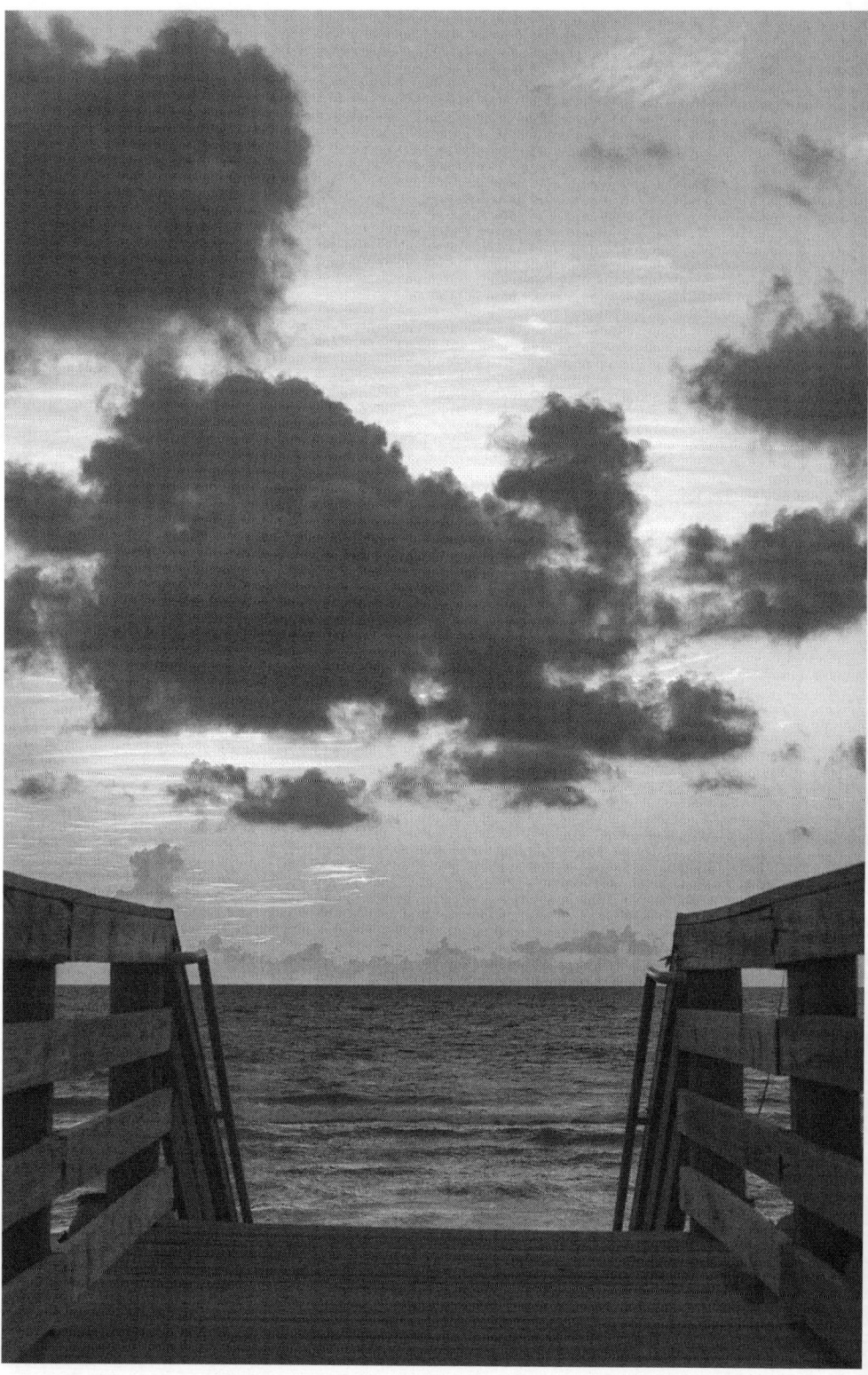

Chapter 4: Energetics & Essence of Nidra

"Relaxation does not mean sleep. Relaxation means to be blissfully happy; it has no end. I call bliss absolute relaxation; sleep is a different matter. Sleep gives only mind and sense relaxation. Bliss relaxes the ātma, the inner self; that is why, in tantra, Yoga Nidra is the doorway to Samādhi."—Swami Satyananda, 1976

Nyasa: Subtle Energy, Inner Focus, and The Guru

Let's introduce the concept of *nyasa* with a dictionary definition. The *Oxford Sanskrit English Dictionary* defines Nyasa as "to place, to set on or in, to use, to touch." Expanding upon that, with some much-needed clarity, the definition also states that Nyasa is "mental consecration or allocation of various bodily parts to guardian spirits." Those are two rather different definitions and fail to properly encapsulate Nyasa, so let's build from there.

Perhaps Agehananda Bharati, a Sanskrit academic and Hindu monk, details Nyasa best. As defined by Agehananda, Nyasa is "the process of charging a part of the body, or an organ of another living body, with a specified power through touch." In Nidra, the touch is from the conscious focus of the mind and not the physical touch of a hand to heart per se, but the energetic exchange remains the same.

In the context of Yoga Nidra, mantras are used or "placed" within a yogi's body with the aid of physical touch. Mantras are chosen phrases, prayers, or affirmations stated repeatedly in the same way you might repeat a poem or a lyric. You would not physically put them anywhere. The idea is that while in a Nidra state, your mind is more receptive, so the mantras can find their way to become more permanent and a part of you in an energetic sense. These mantras aid in elevating one's consciousness and connecting them more readily with their guru or "guardian spirits.: Throughout the duration of Nyasa, lasting a few minutes, a yogi directs their focus and *mentally* touches parts of their body—there is no physical interference. All the while, the mantras are repeated.

The Gheranda-Samhita, a Sanskrit text in Hinduism, contains the following instruction for a yogi: "Next he should place the *guru* etc. [in his body], as instructed by the guru, and commence with the purification of the channels through breath control." The breath control aspect of the quoted material does not relate to Nidra, but the idea of "placing" the guru in the energetic, non-physical body can be linked.

With the guru existing within, and their Spirit dancing with that of the yogi's, bliss and some semblance of enlightenment might become more apparent. Thanks to Nyasa, a yogi can awaken subtle energy, the non-tangible and ethereal essence of Spirit and Divinity, within the physical body. All of these subtle connections occur beyond what can be seen, felt, or physically experienced.

Sādhanā: The Spiritual Spiral

Following up on Nyasa, we have sādhanā. Sādhanā is your daily spiritual practice, and how that looks might be entirely different from one day to another. At first, sādhanā might take up only a minimal amount of your day. As your interest, knowledge, and diligence unfurl, your sādhanā's time and importance will likely grow and expand.

Here are a few key reminders that might aid in cultivating a diligent and beneficial sādhanā:
- Honor yourself—it's your time, after all. If you plan ahead and allow time specifically for your practice, show up for yourself at that moment—in mind, in spirit, and in body. "Making it" to your practice creates some inner turmoil at times, but rarely is there a circumstance where you regret practicing.

- Honor your teachers—respecting others' time stands in high regard within the morals of yoga. Plenty of teachers, myself included, are not thrilled when students pop out of a class prior to savasana and the closing of the class. The cultivation of a class, especially with the sacred nature of Nidra, requires hours of training leading up to the actual holding of space. Remain aware of such time, and honor the work of your teachers by showing up fully and being present.

- Follow the moral guidelines of your chosen path—an abundance of varying yoga styles and philosophy systems exist, some of which might meld with Nidra, while others may not. Either way, most paths carry a moral code of sorts within them. For instance, along the eightfold path, a yogi's ethical guide is found in the Yamas and Niyamas. Shared in the *Yoga Sutras of Patañjali*, the Yamas encourage yogis to *avoid* violence, lying, expelling unnecessary energy, and attachment. The Niyamas invite yogis to *embrace* hygiene and cleanliness, as well as a sense of contentment, purification, and endless studies, then surrender to Spirit energy. Nidra itself exists as a profoundly intimate and internal experience, so your morals are left up to you.

- Stoke the fire—find what thrills you and inspires you within your chosen path or course of study. Within the realm of Nidra, perhaps the idea of Nyasa and mantra stimulates you. Shift your focus to Nyasa for a while and *really* dig into the depths of that material. The firsthand experience is best, so base your sādhanā upon an emphasized study of mantra and Nyasa. Studies slow when enthusiasm dissipates, so follow what sets your heart ablaze.

Furthermore, keep in mind that sādhanā is not one singular thing. It might be your thoughts as you sip your morning mug of coffee or tea. Or sādhanā is how you react to having missed the bus to work. Anything and everything can be sādhanā. The idea that learning never stops goes hand-in-hand with the vastness of sādhanā. In order to *do* this, you need only live with presence, aim to grow and deepen your understanding of your yogic path, and use all the tools you have within to expand your consciousness.

State of Mind

You might wonder, *Where, oh where, does my consciousness go during Nidra?* Such a question is entirely valid. After all, your consciousness is not asleep, and it's not entirely present either. This in-between state is unfamiliar to most of us. The unfamiliar, falling under the infamously daunting and simultaneously alluring concept of "other," that which exists beyond what we can fathom, tends to be left untouched and unexplored. Rarely do we venture to the unknown and think, *Hey, that dark room looks fun and totally safe to explore.* Nidra invites you to expand your awareness into these unknown realms, but it can be a more pleasant experience if you have some insight of the process before getting started.

Nidra folks often talk about "heightened states of consciousness," and the term has come up several times already in this text. This sounds pretty important, but *what* are we blabbing on about? Energetically, heightened states of consciousness are linked to the shift in brain waves mentioned earlier. While your "normal" waking consciousness might think about the more mundane things we humans spend time on, such as eating lunch, taking a shower, providing for loved ones; your "higher" consciousness interacts more with a form of your higher Self.

Your higher Self exists beyond your "ego," the layer of your being that has *wants* more than *needs*. This aspect of Self can communicate clearly with Source energy, also known as "God" or "Spirit." Whatever you want to call it, the higher energy existing outside of the physical realm and body has a more direct relationship to our higher consciousness than our usual waking minds. So when you are awake and making dinner, you are not directly communing with Source. Nidra, though, allows your mind to rest in a space where ego quiets, presence settles in, and your higher Self can speak loud and clear.

Consciousness doesn't ever go away. You aren't flipping a switch "on" and "off" when you practice Nidra. You *are* shifting your brain waves to induce a higher state of consciousness, but your consciousness remains exactly where it always is, resting within your mind and Spirit. When you wander into Nidra, you don't need to have your consciousness on a leash and tug it back upon returning to "regular" programming. Your consciousness is right there within you, it merely wanders deeper and higher within to speak to Self and Source in a more beneficial manner.

Thinking about such matters can often feel as if your mind is melting a bit. Think of it this way: within you there are energetic, invisible hallways, rooms, doors, and windows. Spirit fills these spaces. Through Nidra, you can come to wander these hallways, open doors, and crack the windows open. You might not walk consciously through every step and vividly open each door, but you can float through these spaces all the same. While wandering through these inner, invisible passageways, you are granted closer access to a Spirit energy, whether you are entirely aware of this or not.

Mantra: Sanskrit Prayer

"The present system of Yoga Nidra, which I have devised, enables people who are unfamiliar with Sanskrit mantras to gain full benefits of the traditional nyasa. It can be beneficially practiced by people of any religion or culture."—Swami Satyananda

Mantra means "mind" and "vehicle." The act of repeating a mantra, your affirmation or prayer, can stimulate your mind and begin to awaken your thoughts and energy. Through the repetition of the same words over time, they grow to be something *more* than words. The rhythm and precise meaning to you will impact how they shift your energy.

Earlier, we reviewed how Swami Satyananda initially experienced Nidra thanks to his remembrance of the students' mantras. Originally formed in Hinduism and Buddhism, a mantra has many different uses. In its essence, a mantra is a (typically Sanskrit) word, phrase, or sound repeated to aid in mindfulness during meditation. Mantras hone one's concentration inward and allow for the mind to quiet by drawing focus to the repeated word or phrase.

Mantras carry specific energies and essences within them. When chanted, the energy is projected both into the room or environment where the practice is being held, and within the person chanting.

Below is a list of a few mantras that new practitioners of Nidra might find helpful. You might shift them in their tense or precise language to align them with your present experience and callings.

- *I am awakening my subtle mind and body.*
- *I am consciously uplifting myself and all beings I form connections with.*
- *I will transcend within myself and expand my senses.*
- *I will slowly channel Divine energy so as to move in tune with natural rhythms.*

Later on, we can explore mantras a bit more through the creativity stimulated in Nidra and the last few phases as you explore a 21-day Nidra guide.

Samskaras: Universal DNA

The shifts occurring through breath awareness, mantra repetition, and visualization cannot be entirely conceptualized within your mind. Our minds do have some constraints, as you likely know. Have you ever thought *really* hard, focused all your might on a concept—the vastness of the universe and what might live beyond—but you find yourself straining to fathom such unfamiliar concepts? The work you are doing through Nidra exists in a similar way. You cannot totally see and witness the transformational work.

Unlearning, relearning, and reprogramming can be entirely invisible to you in the physical sense. It might show up minimally throughout your day when you are less reactive in stressful situations and find your breath and balance with greater ease, or it might never show itself to you. But it's there.

Through these methods of mindfulness and repatterning, you are working on the archetypes of the universe—*samskaras*.

What are samskaras? Well, they are a bit difficult to describe due to their ethereal ways, but let's try to unwrap the concept. In essence, Samskaras might be compared to seeds. They are universal symbols that imprint themselves on our minds, and in a sense, upon our very DNA. Alternatively, Samskaras might be likened to the coding language of computer programming, but few can come to learn the coding of the universe. There are no "Samskara scientists" who entirely understand the inner workings. The ancient Yogis who discovered the benefits of repeating mantras are about as close to Samskara experts as it gets.

Samskaras imprint upon you and are inherently within you. They need only be activated, through mantra, breathwork, and other vibrational shifts. Once activated, they can bloom and bud into action. Over time, they grow more and more awake and energized to release their coding within you. The more you chant, repeat your Sankalpa, visualize, and practice Nidra, the more Samskaras are able to continue to unfurl and fully grow.

The shifts in coding will not actually affect your DNA but can affect your habitual behaviors, thought patterns, and personal growth. If you have been feeling stuck in a cycle of behavior and it feels as if you have dug yourself a deep, grooved hole, Samskaras lift you up. They fill in the grooves and make it difficult for you to return to what once was. They can uplift your overall energy so that you no longer feel compelled or entirely able to return to bad habits or intrusive, negative thoughts.

Chakras: Subtle Energy Channels

In many ways, Nidra becomes a balancing act between the space of consciousness and sleep, between natural thought and mantra, between sensation and ethereal space. Chakras often find their way into a Nidra script or session as they offer a similar balancing act.

Most people have heard of chakras, at least in passing. Their colors and concepts have filled the shelves of metaphysical shops for ages, with prints, tapestries, crystal decor, and the like—sharing their essence. The main chakras are known fairly well by most yogis nowadays. The chakras which exist beyond your physical body might be unfamiliar. I know I had *no* idea up until a few years ago that there are chakras beyond the ones dancing about my physical being.

In Sanskrit, Chakra translates to "wheel." Your chakras are spinning energy centers, typically aligning themselves with the midline of your body—the spine. The main chakras are thought to be located in the following places:

Muladhara—*Root*: Very base of the spine
Swadhisthana—*Sacral*: Between belly button and Root, near the pubic bone
Manipura—*Solar Plexus*: Center of the chest, near the sternum
Anahata—*Heart*: Level with the heart, but rests at the center of the chest
Vishuddha—*Throat*: Base of the throat
Anja—*Third Eye*: Space between the brows
Sahasrara—*Crown*: Top of the skull

Each chakra contains unique energy. At all times, they are in communication with one another in some way or another. As they are "wheels," spinning and turning within, a constant give and take of energy occurs. If this give and take features any imbalances, you might experience a blockage or feel *too* open within that chakra and its essence.

You can study and connect with your chakras to bring them into balance. Imagine an old-fashioned balance scale, with two plates that must be perfectly balanced by the pressure placed upon each plate. There will be constant adjustment in order to maintain perfect balance. Balancing your chakras might be an endless dance in many ways. Working with your energy takes time to understand, and *controlling* your energy takes even longer. You might balance your Root chakra, but realize that upon doing so your Crown chakra now feels blocked. Balance is a dance, an endless walk, and one ripe with opportunity for the curious and the wild.

The energetics of the "main" chakras vary from person to person, but the main essence stands. Here are the typical energies and concepts linked to each chakra:

Muladhara—*Root*: Grounding, stability, stillness, Earth
Swadhisthana—*Sacral*: Sexuality, desire, pleasure, vitality, Lunar, Fire
Manipura—*Solar Plexus*: Sense of Self, will power, joy, Fire
Anahata—*Heart*: Compassion, kindness, love, interconnectedness, Water
Vishuddha—*Throat*: Communication, voice, creative expression, Water
Anja—*Third Eye*: Intuition, psychic nature, insight, Air
Sahasrara—*Crown*: Bliss, awakening, intuition, understanding, Air

Through an exploration of your specific chakras, you might come to better know your energetic and subtle body. Your energy extends beyond the spinning thresholds of the chakra system, but gaining the insight and balance others have already gathered can guide you deeper within your own understanding. With some knowledge to carry, forging ahead into the unknown and unfamiliar might be a bit more comfortable.

Exploring Samadhi and The Cutting of Ties

Samadhi can be defined as a state that can be reached over time through the practice of yoga and similar spiritual practices. When translated, Samadhi means "to direct together." Pronunciation is as follows: *sah-mah-tee*

With Hindu and Buddhist roots, it relates to the union of an individual's soul with the infinite spirit. Through Nidra, one can make their way toward this state. Within Samadhi, a yogi can clearly see how their identity is not physical but composed of Spirit, Source, and Divine. Human consciousness heightens to a state where it can merge and become entirely one with cosmic consciousness. A yogi can fully conceptualize how they exist beyond the physical body.

There are two phases involved in Samadhi. The first phase is *sabikalpa*, where a yogi or meditator experiences their essence melding entirely with spiritual consciousness and its infinite source energy. But, once meditation closes, Samadhi ceases as well. You cannot bottle up this connection or carry it with you outside of the moment. It's a release of delusion in some ways but is impermanent. The spirit of the yogi remains bound to the ego and conscious thought.

The second phase is *nirbikalpa*. During this stage, unconditioned oneness occurs. Sabikalpa was *conditioned* oneness. In *nirbikalpa*, ego restraints dissipate. As a yogi or meditator releases, they are endlessly in union with God, Spirit, Source energy. The delusion of separation from God does not return after *nirbikalpa* as it would following *sabikalpa*. Nirbikalpa requires work and asks one to explore their ties to ego and worldly attachments. Through confrontation and introspection, one can work through the release and cut ties with worldly thought and desire.

Samadhi is often misinterpreted to be entirely linked with death and the act of leaving one's body. Such is not the case, as that is one "form" of Samadhi. MahāSamadhi is the act of leaving one's body with intention, fully detached from vessel and mind. It is the final form of Samadhi and arrives when a yogi reaches an enlightened state and chooses to detach. There are notable differences between this act of dying and the physical death of an unenlightened person.

Paramhansa Yogananda, an Indian yogi and guru, wrote a poem called Samadhi which details a yogi's experience in Samadhi. The language used might be beneficial during the visualization phase of your Nidra practice. Alternatively, it could aid in your cultivation of a Sankalpa. Here is an excerpt from Yogananda's *Samadhi*:

I swallowed, transmuted all
Into a vast ocean of blood of my own one Being!
Smoldering joy, oft-puffed by meditation,
Blinding my tearful eyes,
Burst into immortal flames of bliss,
Consumed my tears, my frame, my all.

Samadhi but extends my conscious realm
Beyond the limits of the mortal frame
To farthest boundary of eternity
Where I, the Cosmic Sea,
Watch the little ego floating in me.

Some aspects of the experiences Yogananda shares in *Samadhi* sound familiar to the manifestation of opposites (more on that to come) that one experiences in Nidra. In other ways, his language could be used during the visualization phase of Nidra. The poem in its entirety shares further experiences that could work to validate your experiences in your Nidra practice.

The Nadis: Nerves & The Subtle Body

Within you, there are three main forms of prana shakti, or "pranic energy." They flow through all you are, similar to our physical nervous systems. Through methods such as mantra repetition and breath awareness, as practiced in Nidra, you can shift the flow of life force energy, otherwise known as *prana* or *pranic energy*. Your physical body, the sacred vessel carrying you through your earthly days, is carried by the pranic energy field. It nourishes and maintains your body's life force and energy.

The three Nadis I'll be speaking about are Ida, Pingala, and Sushumna. Nadis carry prana, *life force energy*, within them, but do so in different ways.

1. Ida—Dancing with Pingala and acting in duality, Ida is the moon. The realm of Ida consists of sleep, dreamland, and the inner, often unseen, workings of your mind.
2. Pingala—Working "opposite" Ida, Pingala is solar, awake, daylight, a realm of growth and energizing activity. Both Pingala and Ida are meant to be in balance.
3. Sushumna—Sushumna takes things up a notch as it acts as a neutral energy, existing outside of the light and dark of Ida and Pingala. Sushumna is a realm of balance and equanimity through prana shakti. You dance with Sushumna during meditative states as your nervous system finds a state of calm and you rest in a sort of in-between state.

Through the control of prana, most likely practiced through some form of pranayama, you can shift your pranic body and flow. You can come to better know this life force energy through your nose. That's right, your nose is a lot more mystical than you might have imagined.

Ida relates to the left side of your body. Pingala relates to the right side. You can determine which Nadi is more "in control" or "dominate" at present by noting which of your nostrils feels more open. If you track the state of your sinuses for a bit, you might come to see that the dominant nostril is always switching. One moment, you can breathe better through the left side. An hour later, your right nostril is clear and the left proves to be a bit congested.

Sushumna arrives on occasion. It is experienced as equally free-flowing breath through both nostrils, or as a momentary pause where no breath flows at all. Such balance is Sushumna, as no clear dominance presents itself in your physical body.

Through studying prana, widely and within yourself, you can come to better understand your pranic flow. At any given moment, you can tap into your breath and feel which Nadi is dominant. It allows you an insight into your present state at the level of the subtle body that might be otherwise unclear to the conscious, everyday mind.

For instance, if you cannot fall asleep at night and are growing increasingly frustrated, you might be in a state where your subtle body and nervous system feel as if they should still be fully up and running. Notice your breath. Plug one nostril and then the other. Which is more congested or has less flow? Chances are, your right nostril feels a bit more open, so the Pingala Nadi is still up and running. With its solar energy, your deeper levels of being are still fully "on" even though your physical body is craving rest. Through a brief pranayama practice or a quick Nidra session, you can bring your Ida Nadi into play and invite in the lunar waves of sweet sleep.

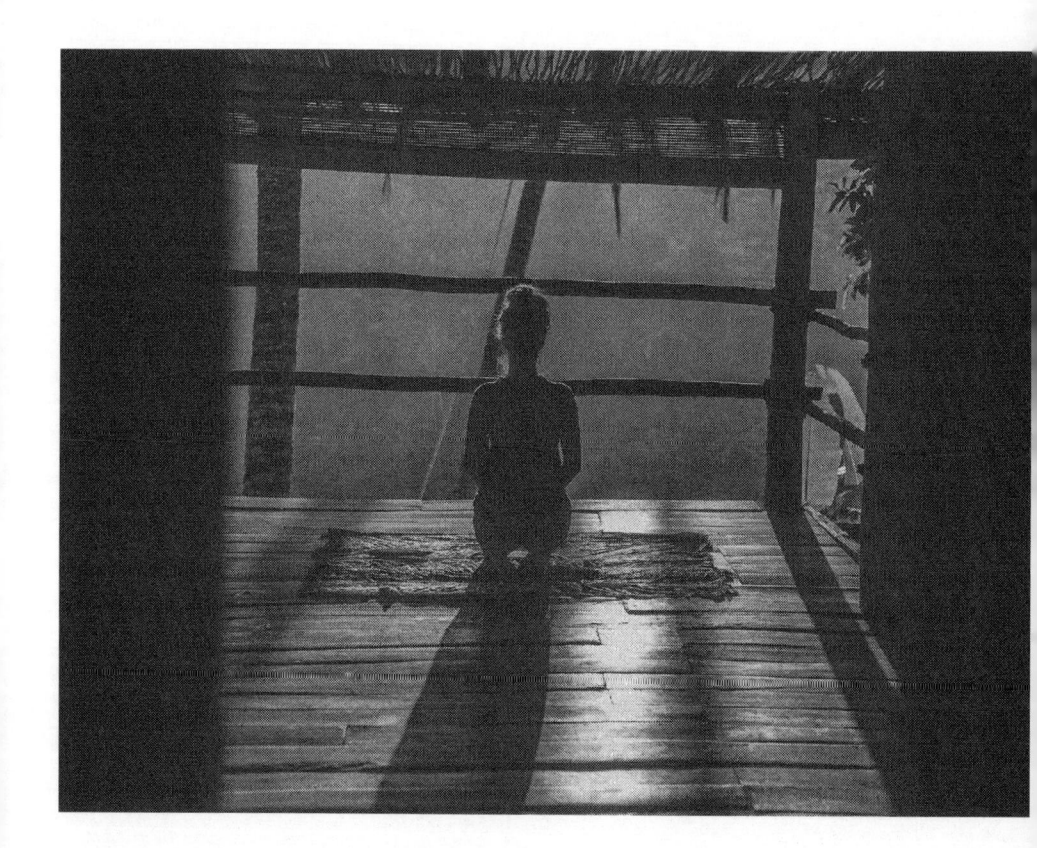

Here is a sort of a "cheat sheet" to sum up the concepts of the Nadis:

Ida's essence:
- Ease
- Spirals around the Sushumna Nadi
- Begins and ends on left side
- Lunar
- Cool
- Nurturer
- Loving-Mother-energy
- Feminine energetics
- Dreamy
- Sleepy
- Mental

Pingala's essence:
- Wild
- Spirals around the Sushumna Nadi
- Begins and ends on right side
- Warm
- Solar
- Protector
- Diligent-Father-energy
- Masculine energetics
- Awake
- Reddened
- Somatic

Through their subtle dance, Ida and Pingala create an elixir between the following:
- Intuition and rationality
- Consciousness and power
- Feminine and masculine energetics

The most potent way to bring Ida and Pingala into balance? *Nadi Shodhana*—alternate-nostril breathing, a pranayama technique. Pranayama is the act of regulating, controlling, or merely observing your breath in order to heighten your consciousness.

To practice Nadi Shodhana, you alternate closing one nostril with a finger or two. While doing so, inhale through the open nostril, then close that nostril and release the other (previously closed) nostril. Exhale from the newly opened nostril. Breathe in through the same nostril. Switch your fingers, closing one nostril, opening the other, and repeat this rhythm for a few minutes. Ideally, you will feel more balanced following Nadi Shodhana as the Nadis found a more steady rhythm for their dance.

Pranayama benefits you at any point in time but can be especially potent prior to asana practice or meditation as it prepares you for movement.

Breath as a Conversation

Awareness of your breath is immensely important. The practice of regulating your breath, *pranayama*, remains popular in most yoga studios and classes, but such control is not featured as prominently in Nidra sessions. Still, the importance of the breath holds steady, and for good reason.

Your breath exists, primarily, as a way for you to keep on living and breathing. Such breathing is involuntary, and it is said that the Divine lingers in actions that are involuntary. The concept of the "Divine" can be likened to "Source energy" or "Spirit" or a "God" of some sort. We all have different words for this perceived higher power. In this context, I'll speak in terms of the Divine. You can replace it with whichever word you prefer.

A conversation with the Divine. *That* is your breath. From the moment you are born, and inhale deeply, perhaps let out a cry, you are filled with *prana*—life. What is life but the Divine filling us with Spirit, Soul, cosmic dust heightened to consciousness? And Nidra invites you to explore such cosmic dust to further awaken your mind and spirit.

Next time your breath feels dull and difficult to connect with, remember you are, in that very moment, conversing with the Divine. The higher power above and within you *is listening*. How are you conversing? What are you saying? What messages are you sending in every *exhale*? And, it goes both ways. The conversation with the Divine is indeed a two-way street. What can you *inhale* from Divinity? What messages are you able to channel?

With your breath as your guide, you might channel a shifted Sankalpa, or experience a more clear vision during your practice. Your breath remains with you always. So, beyond the time spent in a Nidra state or while meditating, circle back to your breath. Allow the breath to be a part of your sādhanā, too.

Meridian Lines

Though a more uncommon method, some Nidra sessions might include information on Chinese Meridian theory. In this type of session, the visualization phase of Nidra will hone in on your meridian lines and guide you through them. You might hear the word "chi" rather than "prana," though they carry the same essential meaning—*life force*.

Similar to your ability to move prana, you can move chi and create major shifts in your body. There are twelve main meridians you might hear about. If you are familiar with Yin Yoga, taught within the context of meridians, these might be somewhat familiar to you.

The Yin meridians are as follows:
1. The arm: lung, heart, and pericardium
2. The leg: spleen, kidney, and liver

The Yang meridians are as follows:
1. The arm: large intestine, small intestine, and triple burner
2. The leg: stomach, bladder, and gallbladder

The premise of Meridian-based Yoga Nidra is that in focusing on the meridians more so than specific body parts, chi shifts and an individual can bring about immense energetic shifts within the realm of their life-force energy. Plus, with an emphasis on the dual nature of "Yin," feminine and lunar, and "Yang," masculine and solar, this specific method might bring you into a clear state of balance.

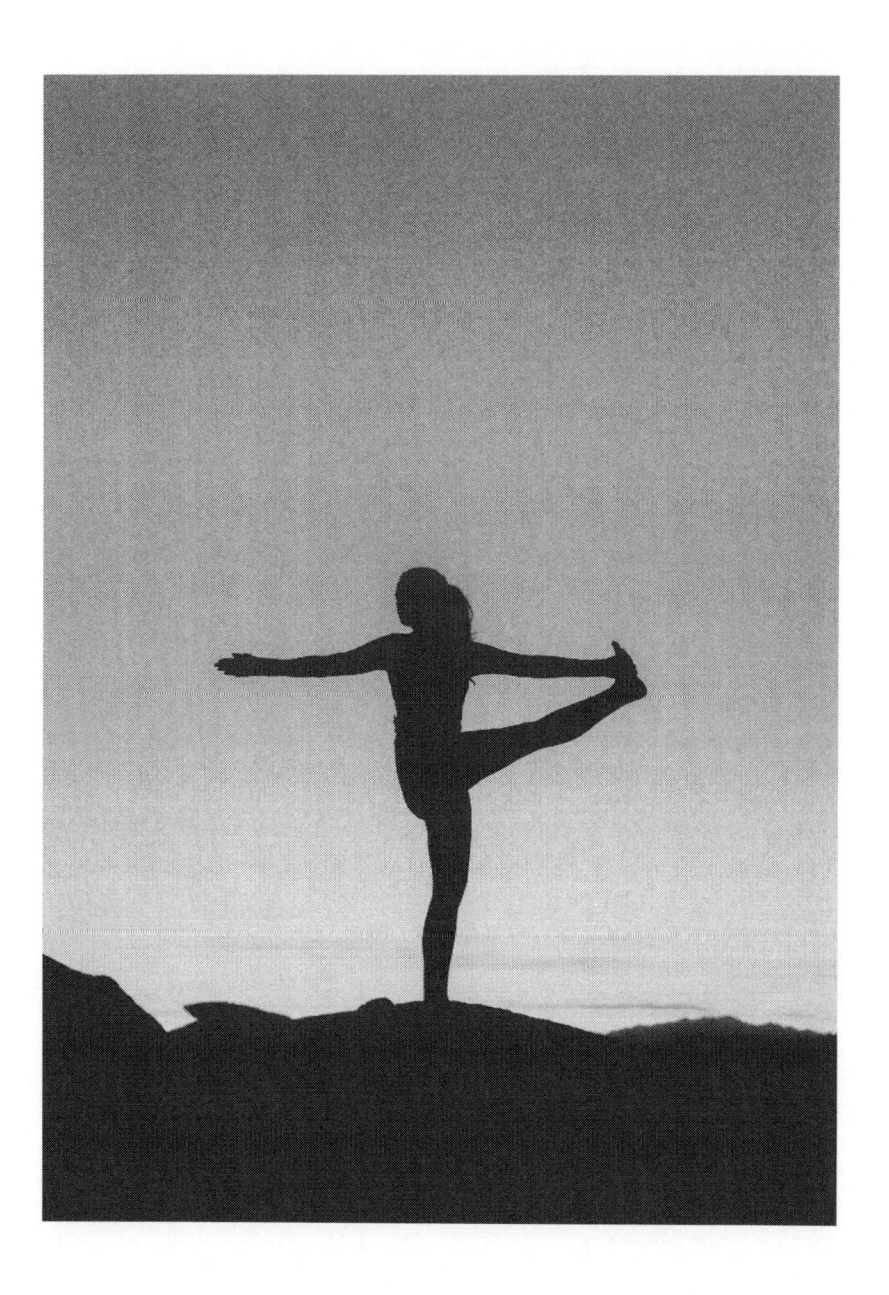

Chapter 5: Benefits of Nidra

The Science in Support of Nidra

Nidra offers peace of mind and acts as an alternative yoga practice for varying individuals and populations. As it is known to be "yogic sleep," the fact that Nidra aids in pacifying chronic insomnia is not surprising. A 2017 study published by Karuna Datta out of *Sleep Science and Practice* shared some specific cases where Nidra was notably beneficial. One patient featured was sixty years old, a widower, and had experienced insomnia for several decades. Another patient was seventy-eight years old, a self-employed business owner, and had complained of insomnia for most of his life. Both patients found that Nidra improved their sleep quality, lowered their depression and anxiety symptoms, and significantly cut back on stress. Researchers checked in with their patients a few months following the treatment, and the improved states of sleep and mental health continued.

Nidra for Women with Menstrual Disorders

Numerous menstrual disorders exist, despite often flying under the radar and rarely coming up in conversation. A 2011 study led by Khushbu Rani was published in the *Industrial Psychiatry Journal* and it explored the efficacy of Yoga Nidra in relation to menstrual disorder patients. Patients were gathered from the Department of Obstetrics and Gynecology at the CSM Medical University in India. One group of females underwent treatment for varying disorders with Yoga Nidra involved, as well as medication. Another group of females only received medication. The first group was receiving Yoga Nidra as complementary medicine, meaning it was provided in addition to conventional methods. The results were incredibly positive—the group receiving Yoga Nidra intervention showed significant improvements in pain symptoms, gastrointestinal symptoms, cardiovascular symptoms, and urogenital symptoms in comparison to the singular medicine group. The researchers concluded that "Yoga Nidra appears to be a promising intervention for psychosomatic problems." What does this mean? In sum, Nidra not only benefits a yogi's mind but their body too.

At present, women's health studies are gaining attention, and discoveries are being made like never before. Due to this increase in medical studies, coinciding with a blossoming of Eastern methods, such as Nidra, alternative and complementary methods are being woven in more readily than what once would have been palatable for Western society. A systematic review which dug into the details of numerous randomized controlled trials, was published in *Complementary Therapies in Clinical Practice*. Conducted by Sang-Dol Kim in 2017, this study assessed the impact of Yoga Nidra on psychological symptoms in women with menstrual disorders. The study supported positive evidence endorsing Yoga Nidra as a treatment for women working to improve their mental health. Most studies seemed to primarily show that anxiety and depression levels were lessened in menstrual disorder patients when adding the practice of Yoga Nidra to their lives. When getting to know your physical body, Nidra offers a soothing approach, rather than an analytical one. Perhaps such lightened ways allow individuals to connect more deeply with their bodies and find healing through that.

Improving women's mental and general health has been significantly lacking until recent years. Studies which explore the possibility that Eastern philosophies such as Nidra might be beneficial to women experiencing pain, illness, and disease are incredibly hopeful. Studies such as Rani's might pave the way for further research on the connection between Nidra, the nervous system, brain waves, and women's reproductive and general health.

Nidra's benefits extend beyond that of the physical. Some of the most magical benefits of Nidra step into a territory that is more metaphysical than tangible and measurable in a research setting.

Generally, Nidra claims the following benefits:

- Deepened awareness
- Opened doorways within
- General healing & rejuvenation

How such benefits arise in a yogi's practice vary from one individual to another. Some folks might experience more benefits in the *externalization* process. There might be more presence and awareness in their days, but less introspection and wandering within. Other folks might be just the opposite. It's common to feel incredibly grounded and receive the outer world with clarity while still feeling called to explore the mind and energetic body more than usual. Regardless of the sensations associated with the experience, the benefits of Nidra affect most practitioners deeply, and the science behind such effects relates primarily to the human nervous system.

Studying the realities of Nidra's ability to "open doorways within" extends beyond that of measurable and quantifiable means. Who is to judge an individual's personal journey within and its truth, benefits, and connection to Nidra? Such a connection is entirely subjective but has been shared by enough Nidra yogis as a benefit that it remains one of the most explored and attractive benefits of the practice.

Nidra & Your Nervous System

In relation to Nidra, the human body connects to two different states of your nervous system. The Parasympathetic Nervous System (PSNS) is most active during relaxed states such as those experienced in Nidra. The Sympathetic Nervous System (SNS) runs wild when an individual experiences stress or reacts to something in their mind, environment, or interaction. The high paced ways of modern culture shift most individuals into a state of stress response. Now, more than ever, we are forced to remain in a mental and emotional state of being that puts us on edge. Falling into a soothing state where the PSNS can relax and allow your body, mind, and Spirit to do the same is increasingly rare. Nidra is one of many methods that allow the PSNS to work its blissful magic, and this practice is only growing in its necessity.

As society continues to expand its technological connectivity and schedule-worshipping ways, finding time for your PSNS to activate is a must. Otherwise, your wellbeing takes a massive hit and your stress might lead to burnout and anxious tendencies. Nidra slowly cracks away at the mountains of stress built up in your being. Through the practice of quieting the mind, honing in on a Sankalpa, and deepening general awareness, Nidra allows individuals to explore a heightened state of consciousness that will only grow over time.

Nidra & Sleep Disorders

Meditation methods, such as Nidra, have been shown to boost melatonin. Considered a heroic hormone, melatonin—produced in the pineal gland—peaks just before bedtime. Melatonin might also aid in preventing cancer, boosting immunity, slowing aging, and preventing numerous diseases. A study from Rutgers University in 2011 showed that melatonin levels in meditators were boosted significantly compared to that of individuals not meditating. Next time, instead of consuming a tablet of melatonin, you might wish to turn to Nidra for similar results.

Our days were once guided by the light, and come night, we went to bed. This practice has shifted with the harnessing of electricity and technological progress. We have light throughout the night and can comfortably stay up late, even if our bodies and minds desperately crave sleep. Falling into a rhythm similar to that of the Earth's can be incredibly beneficial for your overall health. Granted, you may not be able to go to bed at 4 p.m. during the wintertime, but slowing down through the likes of Nidra might massively shift your rhythms and allow ease to find its way into your days. Nidra invites a sense of balance back into your days (and nights).

Brain Chemicals On Nidra

Known for its contribution to happiness, serotonin seems to be increased during meditation methods such as Nidra. Serotonin, a neurotransmitter, impacts the brain more than most other elements. Positive feelings, such as happiness, are associated with a lower experience of stress, and can notably affect an individual's overall health and well-being. University of Montreal researchers (Perreau-Linck et al.) found that mindfulness practices impact the production of serotonin levels. Mindfulness meditations seem to wash over neurons with the happy waves of serotonin. With the recalibration of serotonin, the brain can also produce new brain cells more productively.

Cortisol, the chemical produced when we are stressed, is often overproduced. Modern humans tend to exist in a "fight or flight" state more often than a "rest and digest" state, causing cortisol to build over time. Mindfulness, along with other alternative medicine treatments, seems to be able to drastically reduce cortisol levels. Cortisol is not only related to stressful conditions, but its constant flooding of the brain can lead to depression, high blood pressure, brain fog, sleep disturbances, overall inflammation, and quickened physical aging.

DHEA, perhaps lesser known than cortisol and serotonin, is a hormone often referred to as the "longevity molecule." Through each passing year, as we age, DHEA production decreases causing aging and disease to accelerate. Mindfulness, Nidra included, can boost DHEA significantly.

Lastly, let's talk endorphins. You might have experienced them while running, also known as a "runner's high," but you can also experience the rush of endorphins through meditation. This natural high might be the "bliss" you feel after a Nidra practice. These neurotransmitters are a natural painkiller and can come about during meditation.

Uplifting Young Folks

Nidra might help in boosting young girls' confidence. Jaspal Kaur Sethi conducted a study in 2013, which was later published in the *Journal of Education and Health Promotion*, assessing the "attention and self-esteem in girls undergoing Integrated Yoga Module." The Integrated Yoga Module (IYM) included methods similar to that of Nidra—Zen meditation, "relaxed alertness," pranayama, Vedic chanting, Yoga asana, and more.

By the end of their research, the girls showed improvement in their attention span, self-esteem, and overall mental health. The researchers made a note that the implementation of similar methods, such as Yoga, counseling, and social support, could drastically improve the girls' state of mind and wellbeing.

Nidra as Complementary Medicine

Nidra often takes a role as *complementary medicine*, meaning patients undergoing typical Western treatment methods might use Nidra in addition to their usual medications. Undergoing treatment, especially within modern medicine techniques, can put a person and their body under immense amounts of stress. Plus, such stress can build up and lead to further issues, such as loss of sleep or heightened anxiety. Thankfully, Nidra offers a sustainable and subtle method of healing. In some cases, Nidra takes on a role in modern medicine as a way to balance one's treatment plan.

Modern treatment and technological advancements have their benefits, though. In 2018, The State University in Copenhagen utilized a PET scanner to further analyze brain activity during Nidra. The information mentioned earlier regarding shifts in brain waves as a result of the practice was discovered in the hospital's research.

The measurements, recorded as EEG, showed that study participants were in a state similar to that of deep sleep for the *entire* Nidra session once guided into the depths. On all electrodes, theta activity rose. Alpha activity showed a reduction, but not in a significant manner. But such insignificance shows that there is a difference between Nidra and sleep. If Alpha waves shifted as they did during sleep, then Nidra's claims of resting in the liminal space of being might be faulty. Thankfully, the PET scanner and modern research backed up the realities of Nidra.

On another interesting note, and in support of the Nidra claim *many* cherish, the same study found that a Nidra state saturates the entire brain and increases dopamine by a significant amount. That bliss you feel post-practice? It's not placebo, nor entirely "woo woo." It's grounded in science, and as time goes on, it is likely that science will continue to prove the benefits of Nidra.

Complementary Healing Method For Cancer Patients

In tune with the idea of releasing stagnant energy and repressed energy, which can be beneficial to almost everyone, Nidra is effective in relieving cancer patients. Through the awareness heightened in Nidra, willpower grows. One can better practice "tapas," or discipline, which might aid in a cancer patient's maintenance of hope.

Throughout any long term healing path, endurance is not only required physically but mentally and emotionally. By growing to better know their mind, a patient can break habitual cycles which might not aid in their healing. Habitual cycles are natural, but often go unnoticed. Nidra brings them right in front of our faces and encourages a gentle confrontation.

Management of Chronic Pain

Chronic pain runs deep, as those who have experienced it are well aware. Beyond physical pain, it can affect an individual's mental, emotional, and spiritual wellbeing. Due to such immense shifts, one's entire life is impacted. Individuals often turn to alternative and complementary medicine as it offers them relief in addition to or in place of conventional medicine. As chronic pain lasts beyond usual periods of healing, a medicine that is equally long and permeating is required. Nidra offers such benefits.

Within the entire realm of chronic pain, Nidra especially benefits neuropathic pain. Neuropathic pain, according to a 2010 *Indian Journal of Palliative Care* article written by Nandini Vallath, "is caused by nerve damage proximal to the sensory nerve endings in the skin." Such pain carries "significant sensory and emotional burdens." In treating neuropathic pain, Yoga Nidra's visualization methods, as well as body and breath awareness, seem to benefit individuals.

Nidra might aid in treating those experiencing cancer pain, too. The visualization shared in Nidra seemed to "sublimate the suppressed emotional components," according to the article from Nandini Vallath, of the body-mind pain connection. Nidra was able to induce sleep and reduce general fatigue in some individuals. Patients experiencing pain—chronic or due to treatment—tend to have difficulty sleeping, so during waking hours, they tend to feel sluggish.

Through the melding of mind and body in Nidra and other meditative, pranayama-based practices, a "dissolution of body" occurred. In losing some sensory awareness and attachment to the body, patients stepped into a more radiant space, ideal for healing. Some patients showed improved self-understanding, acceptance, altered perspectives on pain (for the better), and felt more in control of their lives. Overall quality of life improved through the meditative and connective nature of Nidra.

While discussing "quality of life," Gap Theory is worth mentioning. The Gap Theory concept maintains that the discrepancy between one's expectations of a given situation and their actual perception can relate to the quality of life. The larger the gap between expectations and actual "reality," the lower the quality of life. Alternately, greater quality of life is perceived when there is a small gap between expectations and reality. Yoga's methods, Nidra included, offer an awareness which then brings expectations and reality into balance. Nidra allows for a deepened overall awareness, so in being more present, you can fully experience the "truth" from your sliver of perceived reality. Plus, yoga encourages practitioners to release expectations. It's hardly a stretch to see a connection, beyond that of scientific evidence, between a smaller gap and the non-attachment and awareness channeled through Nidra.

Thanks to the means of modern medicine and technology, Nidra has the space to transcend its present state and only grow in its efficacy. With its many benefits, Nidra stands a chance in transforming modern medicine and taking on a more powerful role as an alternative healing method. Nidra can act as an alternative therapy in some cases, perhaps offering healing to those experiencing anxiety, PTSD, or depression who do not wish to abide by conventional methods. Or, Nidra can offer complementary healing remedies to those who enjoy conventional medicine but wish to explore every option out there.

For now, Nidra—acting as complementary medicine—is a much-needed step forward. The melding of Eastern and Western philosophy has occurred on a minor level in recent decades. In many ways, Eastern philosophies and culture have been appropriated. While this is certainly a reality, proper conversation and respectful research and discourse allow us to unpack assumptions from reality. With that, Nidra and other Eastern practices can take a more natural and honored stance in our Western days and ways.

Common Questions Asked & Answered

Can I practice Nidra and skip "regular" sleep?

The short answer here: *No.* Sleep is a period of *pure* rest for almost every aspect of your being. Nidra isn't too far off from this state, but the awareness maintained within your consciousness differs from the way the brain quiets during deep sleep. While you might feel incredibly rejuvenated after practicing Nidra, perhaps sometimes more so than your usual night's rest, it should not be used as a means of skipping sleep entirely. Of course, if you suffer from sleep disturbances, insomnia, or something of the sort, Nidra might take on a more significant role in your sleep. What would I *not* recommend? Skipping out on a good night's rest right before an exam or presentation, and counting on Nidra to make up for the loss. Your practice likely looks and feels different *every* day. What if the *one* day you choose to use Nidra as a means of catching up on your eight hours is the same day your practice isn't as present and depth-filled as usual?

Why shouldn't I fall asleep during Nidra?

Drifting off to sleep during meditation is incredibly common when you're just beginning to dip your toes into the practice. Similar sleepiness arises during Nidra, especially if you have not had your usual eight hours of true sleep as of late. Catching up on sleep during your Nidra practice, though, is far from the point. Nidra allows you to rest in a space between sleep and proper consciousness, so avoiding sleep is key. Of course, if you have had some late nights lately, drifting off is sometimes a bit too tempting for the body. Combat this desire by inviting some diligence into your Nidra practice, inviting a balance between relaxation and presence.

Within the realms of Daoist thought and theory and various other philosophy systems, the ideas of *Mother* and *Father* energy exist. Mother energy appears as loving, nurturing, gentle, and fluid. Father energy shows up as a bit more rigid, with high expectations and a more demanding presence calling for respect. You might explore these two energies within your practice. At which point can you call in some Mother energy and treat yourself with a gentle openness? When your mind falls to the wayside and thoughts begin to spiral, or you find yourself skipping several days of practice in a row, Father energy might benefit you.

With that in mind, carry some diligent Father energy into your Nidra practice if you notice you tend to drift off into full-on sleep. The stoicism of the Father energy can encourage you to remain present in the Nidra state, no matter how badly you crave a moment of pure sleep.

Again, though, if you are in need of catching up on your sleep, Nidra can be a way to supplement your disrupted sleep schedule and help you catch up a bit quicker. But such a replacement should be used scarcely and only when entirely necessary.

How can I stay alert during Nidra?

Drifting off to dreamland more often than you might like? Here are a few mindfulness techniques to keep your mind in check (more will be outlined in the 21-day challenge, as well).

- Counting: A simple method, in theory, but acts as a great practice in presence. When you focus on your breath during Nidra, *count* the seconds for every inhale and exhale. Perhaps you inhale for a count of five, exhale for a count of five. To build upon this and *really* keep your mind and presence in check, also track how many cycles of breath you experience in your practice. You might end up counting higher than you would expect. Treating this method like a gentle game can make it a bit more engaging.

- Envision: With every inhale, imagine a wave crashing over the thoughts in your mind. As you exhale, the wave draws itself back out to sea. Any intrusive thoughts or inklings beyond that of your Sankalpa are drawn out with the sea. So, to reiterate: Inhale, waves crash onto your mind. Exhale, waves pull back out to sea and take your wandering thoughts along for the ride.

- Embrace: Grant yourself a moment. Allow your thoughts to dance about as they would like. Perhaps, some thoughts rise to the surface and stimulate your entire being for a moment. Thereby, you are able to walk away from dreamland for a bit. A gentle approach soars above that of an aggressive or frustrated one. Let your thoughts simply be for a moment. This acts as the equivalent of letting a toddler express their tantrum for a moment. Or, a deep sigh of relief, but for your mind alone. Embrace the mess. It's what so many folks are experiencing, too, so don't beat yourself up about it. Allow space for your mind and breath to return to center. Patience is your guide here.

- Deepen: Breathwork affects humans on a cellular level. If you would like to quiet your nature for a moment, deepen your exhale. Exhales act as a potent release when lengthened. Inhales move in the other direction. Lengthen your inhale if you would like to wake up a bit. Breathe deeper into your low belly and hips, perhaps even sending your breath toward the crown of your head to shift your focus and stir your mind. Remain with lengthened inhales until you feel a smidge less sleepy.

Is Nidra like hypnosis?

No, your teacher will not make you act wild and crazy during your time between wake and sleep, as you might have seen in a hypnosis set intended for entertainment. The trance-like state achieved in Nidra finds itself compared to hypnosis fairly often, and in some ways this makes sense. In both states of being, deep relaxation is brought about by the vocal cues of a hypnotist or teacher. The body melts away and the mind remains focused. Nidra *can* be used to influence your mind, but in a different realm of science than hypnosis. In Nidra, you are in control. Your teacher is merely there to guide you in, remind you to remain in your state of meditation, and draw you back out. Hypnotists, whether for "fun" or for psychotherapy purposes, have a more engaged role as they have a goal involved in their process. You are entirely responsible for yourself within the practice of Yoga Nidra. Yoga Nidra invites you to explore your cyclical ways, behaviors, and consciousness. Hypnosis can be used to change your ways and behaviors, but the shifts are fully disclosed and act as a goal for the hypnotist. In Nidra, there is no precise goal in mind, though some sort of healing or behavioral shift might come about.

How can I begin my practice?

Your practice began the moment you stepped toward this path. Now, it's up to you to find your way. Do you feel called to find a teacher in your local community? My recommendation would be to ask around and explore the teacher's messages that can often be found online. Do you align with what they are sharing? Do you think you would be comfortable sharing in the space they are holding? If the answer is a resounding "Yes," then give their classes a try. Even if you don't entirely *love* your first Nidra class, your second, third, or tenth experience might be the turning point for you. If you feel called, continue to show up for Nidra as it reveals its ways to you.

How can I make Nidra accessible for me?

Address your needs. What would make your Nidra practice ideal? What concepts in Nidra are daunting to you? If you feel comfortable doing so, you can share your needs and feelings with your teacher so they can meet you where you are. Experienced teachers always appreciate honesty, openness, and clarity in our teacher-student relationships. We love to hear about your thoughts and feelings, and a respectful teacher will always account for your needs. For example, if you are uncomfortable closing your eyes and resting in total darkness, a teacher should honor that.

If you cannot lay down for extended periods of time, a teacher should make other options work for you and share those options with you. If you are practicing solo, honor your personal edges. Whether they be physical, mental, or emotional. You know "you" best.

The relaxation brought about in Nidra only arrives if you are resting comfortably and feel held. Do whatever you need to make that possible. On a day to day basis, your practice might look different. One day, your eyes shut with ease. The next, it's a bit difficult to rest in darkness. Take your practice as it arrives. Honor your ebbs and flows.

Is Nidra for me?

Nidra is for everyone, truly. Whoever feels called to explore Nidra—whoever resists Nidra—we all can come to love the murky waters of this introspective and transformative practice. Of course, you might outgrow your practice. From such growth, you might expand beyond Nidra and never circle back. Or your growth might lead you back to Nidra eventually. Our teachers and lessons arrive in your path during specific times and remain only for as long as they are necessary. See this to be true and allow your relationship with Nidra to unfurl as is intended.

I experienced _____ during Nidra—is that normal?

Unless you experienced physical pain, then *yes*, I'm willing to bet your experience was normal. Did you experience some "trippy" visual effects? Did you feel a crumbling of your ego? A cracking open of your heart (in an energetic sense)? I can tell you I've experienced all of the above more than once. The first time, though, can certainly be jarring. Who knew yoga could be such a trip? This certainly wasn't advertised in the class description.

At any point in time, if you experience something notably heavy or physically uncomfortable, share this information with your teacher or a friend who might be able to hold space for you. Nidra can draw you into spaces steeped in darkness. Our inner realms are no joke! Allowing yourself to experience this level of vulnerability might be daunting, but I highly encourage you to share if you feel the need to "lighten up" following or during your practice. And if you really are not sure if something is "normal," check with someone who might have a direct answer to your specific experience. Questions and curiosity are a natural vine growing along your path.

Do I have to practice vinyasa, or any asana, before yoga Nidra?

Absolutely not! Especially if you don't want to practice asana. Nidra can stand entirely on its own. Sometimes it is offered after asana practice, but that does not mean you need to *always* practice asana first. The intention of asana is to prepare your *mind* and *spirit* for a closing meditation. That's why savasana acts as a bookend to asana classes. Meditation is the entire point. You were always headed there in every single asana class you have ever attended. Nidra is that "end point" expanded and specified to allow more depths and release.

Who can benefit from Nidra?

The following populations and communities have been shown to benefit from Nidra:
- PTSD patients
- Military combat veterans
- Menstrual disorder patients
- Trauma recovery patients
- Individuals with anxiety
- Individuals with depression
- Schoolchildren
- College students

So, that's a lot of different groups with some potential overlapping. Everyone can benefit from Nidra, and that's part of its beauty. The accessibility of Nidra will likely only continue to grow with programs such as iRest (Integrative Rest) aiding in spreading Nidra's benefits.

How should I position myself during Nidra?

How you choose to rest during Nidra is entirely up to you. If reclining flat on your back is not accessible for you, try leaning against a wall. Nidra can be practiced in any setting, and choosing not to recline will not make much of a difference in your practice. As long as you are supported, you can rest however you would like. Keep in mind how relaxation and the "melting" that often occurs during Nidra affect your position of choice though.

If you're looking for support, you can rest blocks underneath your knees. Alternatively, a bolster or rolled up blanket can offer support for your knees. If you tend to feel cold throughout a meditation practice, drape a blanket over your body. The more comfortable you are, the less distracted you're inclined to become.

Can I practice Nidra while laying in bed?

You can practice Nidra wherever you would like. I don't expect anyone to follow you around and berate you for your methods. Be wary of the temptation of sleep, though. Laying in bed might increase your chances of drifting off as your mind likely associates your bed with sleep. If you can stay awake properly while melting into your bed during Nidra, I can't imagine it being an issue.

In some cases, individuals who tend to sit in bed on their laptops or work while cozied up might benefit from bringing the peace of Nidra into the space. Working in bed can then displace the connection between *laying in bed = time to dial my energy down and rest*. Weaving Nidra into the bed could aid in shifting that, thereby granting an individual a proper night's rest.

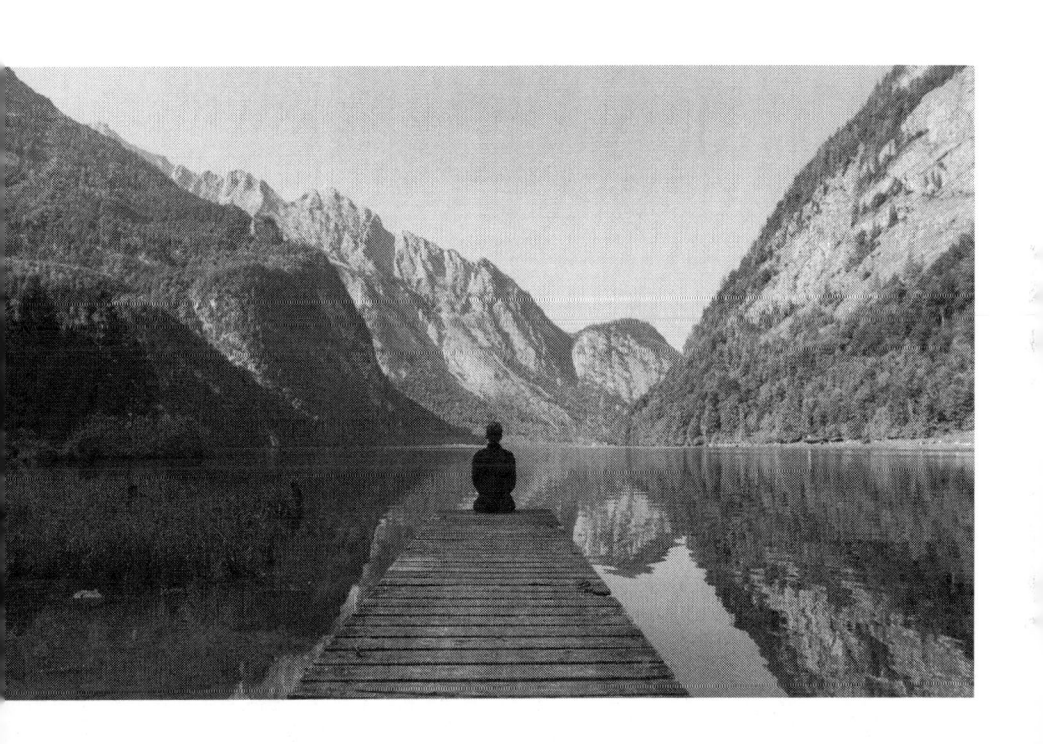

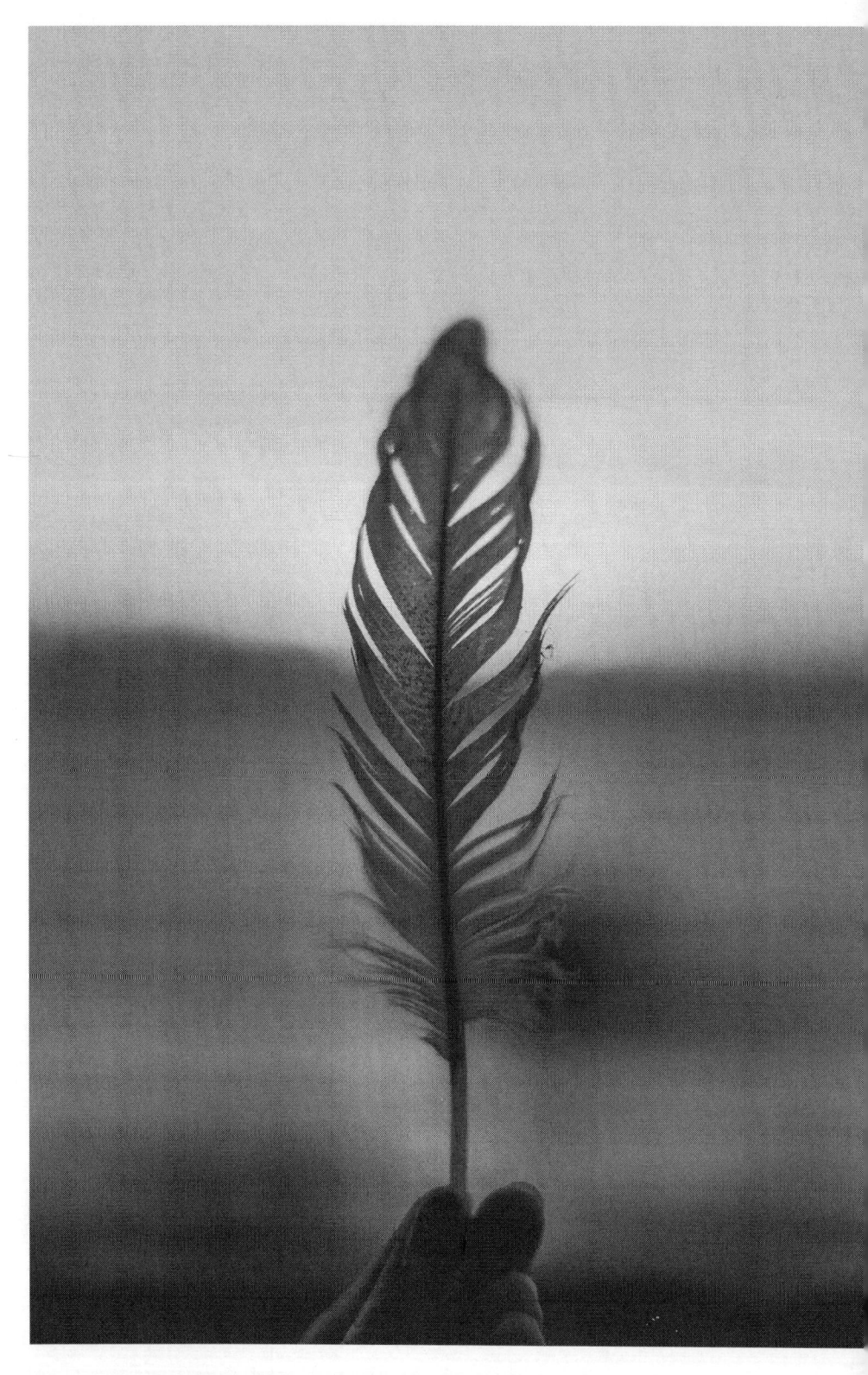

Chapter 6: Scripts of Nidra

The scripts and texts which mention and explore meditation techniques and practices similar to modern Nidra were explored briefly in the earlier history section. They are entirely worth exploring in more detail. After all, they brought Nidra into what it is today and contributed to Swami Satyananda coming to curate present methods.

Earliest References

The following texts will be mentioned, all of which hold their own as *major* texts in varying paths of Eastern religion, culture, and spirituality.

- The Vedas
- The Puranas
- Vijñāna Bhairava Tantra
- Hatha Pradīpikā

You might be wondering why texts which are older than dirt still matter? Well, the contents found in their crumbling pages relates directly to our modern practices. Despite Nidra's recent modernization, it was etched into pages by ancient Indian scholars. If you think about how old that makes this practice, then try to fathom just how beneficial this practice must be if it has remained relevant for so many centuries.

In the *Vedas* and *Puranas*, Nidra is mentioned and discussed. At some points throughout ancient texts, as seen in *Devi Mahatmya, Bhagavata Purana*, we hear of *Vishnu*, a variation of *Shiva*, asleep on the *naga shesha*. What is Vishnu up to? Well, practicing Nidra, of course! Vishnu's practice likely differs greatly from modern Nidra, but the essence remains the same. Vishnu is, after all, the sleeping lord.

In *Mandukya Upanishad*, "prajna" is mentioned and linked to Nidra. *Prajna* refers to the conscious awareness of one's being while in a deep sleep state. Sounds pretty familiar.

Vijñāna Bhairava Tantra

Also referred to as *Vigyana Bhairava Tantra*, this is, as you might have assumed, a major tantra text. Likely written around 800 AD, the *Vigyana Bhairava Tantra* shares wisdom and methods revolving around tantra philosophy and practice.

Within the realm of tantra, the text belongs to Kashmir Shaivism, a specific system. Tantra exists in an ethereal manner similar to Nidra, despite it being a thoroughly studied and practiced philosophy system. Beyond the tangible texts of Nidra, tantra explores the energetics and "whys" of the universe. *Vigyana Bhairava Tantra* was written by Swami Nischalananda Saraswati.

Breaking down the words aids in understanding the purpose and contents of the text. *Vigyana* means "wisdom" and "insight." The word relates to a state of witnessing the world and oneself without forceful thought or labeling of experiences. *Bhairava* means "Shiva," the form of consciousness that bears stoic *Father* energy. Shiva destroys concepts which lead to ignorance, blissful and otherwise, as well as internalized falsehoods or societal expectations.

Stringing the words together, then, creates a more clear picture. The text is a tantra detailing of gaining gentle insight so as to expand and transcend the concepts placed upon us, by our environments, societies, cultures, and others. Methods within tantra, such as Nidra, offer methods that will allow for such potent transformation in a way that will not entirely pull the rug out from under an individual. Perspective is shifted with ease rather than malicious destruction.

Within the *Vigyana Bhairava Tantra* are several concepts which can be linked to modern Nidra. Here are a few, with some of my musings added on.

- **Our innate state of being is Consciousness.** Physicality, perception of outer experiences and environments, and the sensation of energy and matter, are not our most "pure" and central way of being. Higher consciousness, gained through awakening and walking a yogic and/or tantra path, is our nature.

- **112 Techniques are shared in the** Vigyana Bhairava Tantra. All seem to be based on the idea of gathering awareness into one's center through *every* aspect of Sadhana. Washing the dishes, one can dial up their awareness of their mundane task, thereby making the mundane a bit more meaningful. Leading a class, one can dial up their awareness within self even while guiding others. Practicing Nidra, solo or in a group session, one can find themselves with a more present and awakened gaze. The practice of cultivating presence extends beyond the precise timeline of your practice. Sadhana does not stop when the clock strikes 12 and your "obvious" practice closes. The path of awakening runs on endlessly.

- **All of the methods shared throughout the ancient pages exist entirely on their own.** No clear religion or set of morals are ever listed. Such freedom from societal confines emphasizes a common theme in yogic methods—Yoga, tantra, Nidra, and all the magic from these ancient ways, are for all of us. Anyone can honor, practice, and study if they choose.

How did all this wisdom come into being? From what spiritual scholars have gathered, it's thought that Shiva channeled the messages of the *Vigyana Bhairava Tantra* to his wife, Parvati. In a fully receptive state, perhaps opened through Nidra or a similar method, Shiva's messages which would come to be the *Vigyana Bhairava Tantra*, were shared with Parvati. Parvati, walking the path of awakening toward "Truth," heard and experienced such messages enough to be able to share them beyond herself. It is thought that Parvati represents a spiritual seeker on a path similar to yours. Shiva, again, represents consciousness.

Similar to other yogic texts, the *Vigyana Bhairava Tantra* and the scholars who have explored its contents emphasize how Parvati can be all of us. *You* are here, seeking your truth, wandering the murky depths of this path. Your path extends out and saturates every aspect of your being and life. Driving down the road, you have the ability to draw your energy back to center if another driver disturbs you or cuts you off in traffic. With the wisdom of Nidra, breath, and your Sankalpa as your guide, you can channel Divinity through all your days and nights. All actions, reactions, and states of being are open to being a means of awakening.

Hatha Pradīpikā

Nidra is also discussed in the *Hatha Pradīpikā*, detailed by Swami Swatmarama. The *Hatha Pradīpikā* is a major Hatha text, likely written around 1350–1550 AD, or perhaps during the fifteenth or sixteenth century.

Essentially, Hatha consists of *every* yoga asana practice. Despite it being known as a singular specific style within modern times, it technically includes all other styles—Vinyasa, Ashtanga and *all* the rest—including Hot Yoga, Yin Yoga, Rocket Yoga, Forrest Yoga.

Nidra pops up in *Hatha Yoga Pradīpikā*'s fourth chapter. It's only mentioned once, but its inclusion is important as the relevance of the entire text has lasted centuries. Swami Swatmarama seems to have thought that a yogi should practice another yogic technique until yoga Nidra occurs.

The other method to be practiced is known as *Khechari Mudra*. A Hatha practice, khechari mudra can be practiced by curling the tip of one's tongue toward the back of their mouth. Stop the curling once the tongue reaches the space where the nasal cavity, near the uvula, begins. Over time, the tongue becomes *longer* and can achieve this with ease. Mudras are meant to awaken spiritual energies in a yogi's body and each has a specific essence involved. In this case, the mudra is not seen in the fingers or hands. In modern yoga, most popular mudras are practiced safely through the fingers and hands. These methods are merely shared for historical accuracy, but should not be practiced without proper guidance.

Once a yogi arrives in a "state" of Nidra, "Kala" should not exist.
What is *Kala*? Kala bears multiple meanings. In one sense, the word means "black" or "death." Perhaps Swami Swatmarama meant that *death* would not exist. Depending upon your views of death and "afterlife" or rebirth, your interpretation of such might differ from mine or another. Kala also relates to *Dirgha-Kala*, as mentioned in the Yoga *Sutras* shared by Patanjali. *Dirgha-Kala* translates to "long time," and likens itself to the experience of an individual realizing a new path or goal, but will not be purified and completed immediately.

In another realm, *Kala* is a form of Yama, the lord of the underworld. Within Vedic mythology (yes, the same Vedas that created Ayurveda, the lifestyle science of Yoga, and the *Vedas*, ancient Indian texts, curated this as well), Yama was said to be the first human to pass on. Thereby, Yama reigns over the underworld. Again, despite coming from a different realm of thought, Kala connects to destruction.

With all that being said, the *Hatha Yoga Pradīpikā* presents Nidra in a form quite different from its present form. Clearly, many steps were taken which allowed Nidra to evolve into its present state. While you will not achieve *death* through Nidra, it's worth exploring the roots of the present practice. After all, it has come a long way to become its present form.

As it relates to Kashmir Shaivism, *Kala* is mentioned as one of the thirty-six *tattvas*. Tattvas are principles of reality, sort of like the Yamas or Niyamas of the eightfold path in Yoga. Kala exists in a group of tattvas considered *pure impure*. This group details the "soul" and the limitations of a soul. The stage of Kala-tattva occurs when one realizes their limitations, despite bearing a soul. A similarity can be seen here when thinking about *Dirgha-Kala* mentioned above.

In his book, Swami Swatmarama goes on to share the following information on Nidra:

- Nidra intends to quiet your mind
- Nidra intends to declutter your to-do list
- Nidra fills you with Spirit through mantra
- Nidra can lead to a heightened state of being (that sort of clear happiness you might feel after Nidra)
- All you do, beyond Nidra and in Nidra, aid in your awakening
- Exploring your mind and perspective aid in your awakening
- Energetic layers of self can shift about and aid in your awakening
- Worrying about the material world is unnecessary
- Awareness of deeper layers of self, beneath conscious thought, is necessary
- Seeking knowledge in an assertive way is not the way to go about studying yoga and Nidra

The Yamas & Niyamas: An Example of Spiritual Guidelines

For the sake of clarity and proper engagement with these concepts, I'll share some grounded details on the Yamas and Niyamas. While wandering a yogic path, no matter where you stand at present, some guidelines are key. The Yamas and Niyamas offer just that. As you explore Nidra, you might feel inclined to broaden your studies, and the guidelines can aid in such expansion.

There are five Yamas—personal moral guidelines. The first, Sathya, emphasizes truth. One should be truthful in their thoughts, vocal words shared, and actions.

Following Sathya, Ahimsa means "non-violence." Not only non-violence in the general sense of not hurting someone, but practicing non-violence in one's thoughts toward self and others, one's interactions, and one's general action. In not stomping on a bug, one follows Ahimsa. This second Yama asks you to move to a space of peace and love, rather than fear, anger, and the immediate need to react.

The third Yama, Brahmacharya, translates to "conduct consistent with Brahma." While not exactly celibacy, the concept encourages yogis to live in moderation. Overindulgence tends to lead to attachment, which leads to further suffering. Practicing mindful moderation in one's day allows them to follow this Yama.

Astheya, the fourth Yama, is the rather simple concept of non-stealing. One should not take or even "covet," what is not theirs. Jealousy and envy are frowned upon. Again, by not coveting what one does not have, non-attachment comes into play.

Lastly, the fifth Yama, Aparigraha means non-hoarding. Only take as much as you need. If you are out in nature, or shopping in your local grocery store, do not take more than required. Allow for bounty to remain for others. Simplicity and minimalism are key.

Shifting over to the Niyamas, which act as recommended actions and habits, the first is Shouchya. Shouchya relates to cleanliness in body and discipline in one's thoughts, words and actions throughout the day. For instance, if you are in a yoga studio, shouchya might be cleaning up after yourself in shared spaces and arriving with clean clothes and materials.

The second Niyama, Santosha, means contentment. Santosha relates to gratitude—be glad for what you have. In this practice, the mind can quiet and concentrate better.

Tapas, the third Niyama, means austerity. To be austere is to be strict or disciplined. While yoga brings great joy and bliss, one should not become lost floating in such experiences. With that being said, Tapas also does not mean one should practice intensely every single day. More so, Tapas means abiding by your rhythms, honoring your body, and showing up for yourself in an accountable and consistent manner.

Swadhyaya, the fourth Niyama, relates to self-awareness. Through Swadhyaya, one can become more in tune with their unique rhythms. Swadhyaya is practiced through contemplation and introspection, which then leads to varying degrees of realization in relation to one's habits, thoughts, and actions. Swadhyaya connects yogis to the universe; in realizing their rhythms, they come to see how they are connected to all that exists "beyond" their physical body. The popular idea that microcosm shifts lead to macrocosm ripples connects to Swadhyaya.

Ishvara Pranidhana is the fifth and final Niyama. Ishavara Pranidhana translates from Sanskrit to mean "supreme" or "personal God." Its essence is that of dedication, devotion, and surrender to the awareness of divinity.

Recent Texts

Swami Satyananda's book, published in 1976, carries his most potent teachings and experiences. Who better to learn from than the founder himself?

A comprehensive look into the eight stages of Nidra, Nidra's physical healing benefits, the effect on the brain, and the altering of consciousness are included in Swami's writings. Despite the text being a few decades old, it stands as a respected and beneficial resource for teachers and students alike. If you are attending a Nidra teacher training, it might even expand upon the ideas presented within your teachings.

Due to recent revelations, Swami Satyananda Saraswati's actions cannot remain unmentioned in full disclosure alongside his writings and teachings. Sexual abuse allegations were presented to the global yoga community in 2014 and some called for a boycott of Swami's literature.

With a stain upon his lineage, many are unsure how to proceed in their practices, especially as numerous other gurus and teachers fall under similar allegations. Such occurrences should move yogis, both teachers and students, to hold their teachers and elders to a standard which abides by the disciplines shared in the varying styles and philosophies.

No matter how highly regarded a teacher might be, their actions can still fail to be beneficial for students. Hold your teachers accountable for their behavior and methods. If you do not feel comfortable engaging with their teachings and published literature, step away. Your practice and how you go about studying yoga are entirely up to you. There is no harm in removing yourself from a toxic and unsafe space or teacher.

Direct Resources

Below, you can find a compilation of all the texts mentioned above, plus a few other texts relating to the concepts of chakras, mudras, and the like.

Yoga Nidra—Swami Satyananda Saraswati

The Hatha Yoga Pradīpikā—Svātmārāma—Originally printed in Sanskrit

Asana Pranayama Mudra Bandha—Swami Satyananda—Incredible text written with precise details and methods relating to the titular concepts and practices. Beneficial for teachers and students alike.

Vijñāna Bhairava Tantra—Tantric text first appearing in the Kashmir Series of Texts and Studies

The Vedas—Ancient Indian Sanskrit text, Hindu scripture

The Puranas—Ancient religious texts, genre within Indian literature

The Yoga Sutras of Patanjali—Compilation of Indian aphorisms relating to theory and yoga

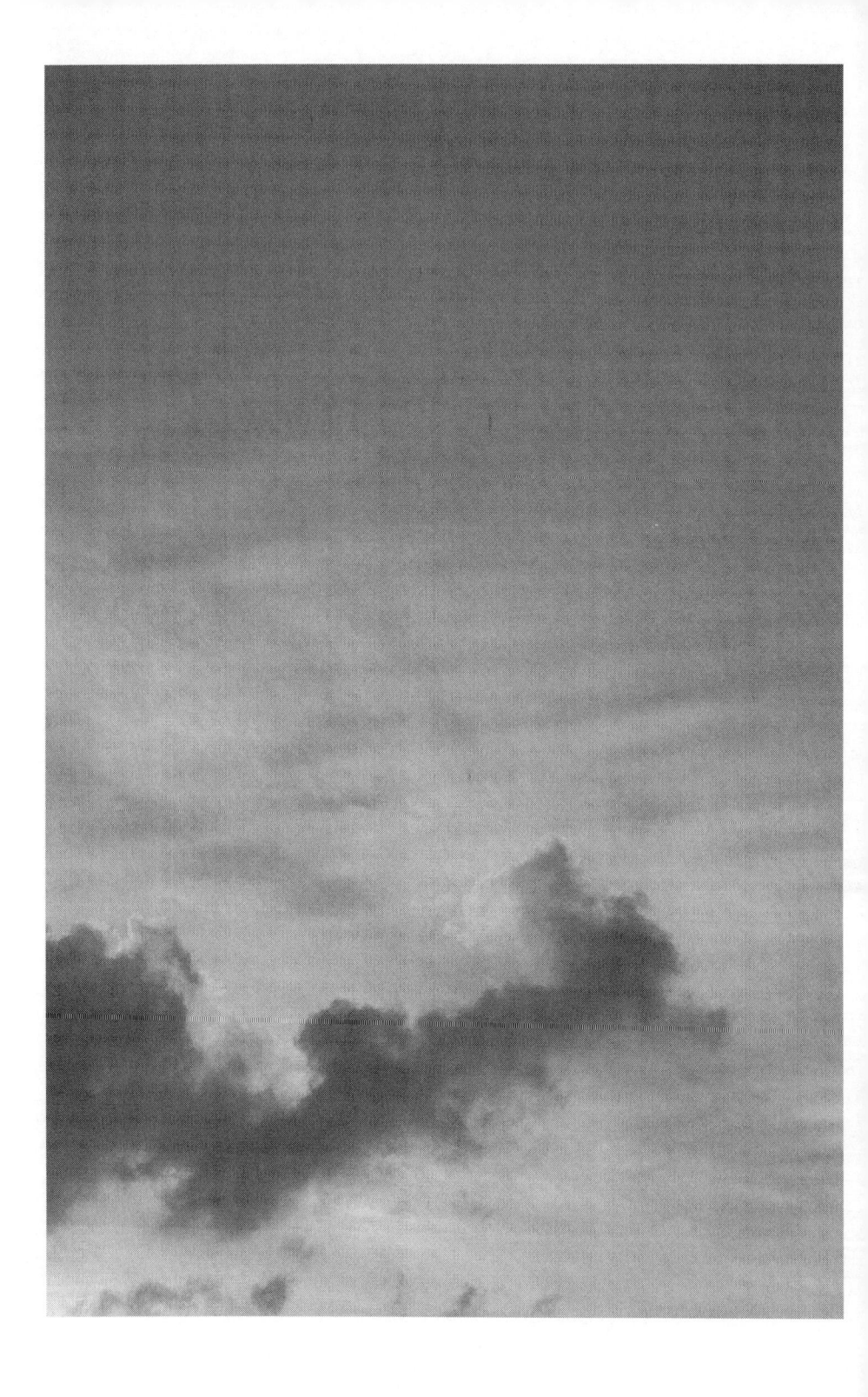

Chapter 7: Build a Personal Practice

Your personal practice entirely coexists with your *sadhana*. Your practice builds itself upon the foundational idea that *all* you do, say, share, experience, and create acts as a means of awakening, teaching, and learning. Your personal Nidra practice acts as a specific method within all this too.

Through the cultivation of a diligent, respectful, consistent, and thorough Nidra practice, you can have a solid main source of *sadhana*. When the spaces in between practice feel as if they are slipping away from you and your learning slows, Nidra can continue to maintain potency.

The yogic paths ebb and flow. One day you might crave a lengthy Nidra session following a brief yoga asana practice, and another day you might find yourself able to rest in Nidra for a shortened period. The best approach to your personal practice instills a sense of non-attachment in all you do.

I'll outline some of the key elements you might include in your practice, physical and beyond, so that you can begin to plant the seeds to become a blossoming and abundant Nidra student.

Combating Negative Self-Talk

When it comes to approaching a new space or taking on something unfamiliar, we tend to allow negative self-talk and doubt to push us away from potential self-growth. Embracing new spaces and ways certainly does not come easy for everyone. But, due to the nature of our minds, we have the power to shift the stories we tell ourselves.

Without realizing it, you might be preventing yourself from stepping into a space of growth and expansion. Even if you are acutely aware of the discomfort in exploring something unfamiliar, you nearly always step out into the "other side" transformed for the better. Embrace the discomfort for a bit. Allow it to guide you further within.

We talk to ourselves endlessly, unless in a meditative state, but even then, thoughts pop up. If you have ever meditated for an extended period of time, you might have noticed the cyclical nature of negative self-talk more than that of positive messages. That little voice in your brain that says *you can't* and *no way*? Yes, most everyone has one of their own. Through the acknowledgment of the falsehoods spoken from that little voice, you can step beyond perceived boundaries. From there, your thoughts no longer hold you back as much as they once did.

Some potential strings of negative thoughts might include the following:

I can't sit still for that long ... Well, I can't imagine *any* teacher berating a student for needing to move a bit, especially a new student. The "rules" of meditation do not have to be as strict as you think. And you could surprise yourself. Nidra's methods are soothing enough to drop even the most rambunctious student into a blissfully calm and still state.

My mind races around too much for that ... Yes, that is why we are all here and return over and over again. Our minds drive us wild, and we *beg* them to slow down. Sadly, begging rarely works. Nidra works wonders though.

I'm not a spiritual person ... Without a doubt, you do not have to consider yourself a spiritual person. No matter your religion or spiritual preferences and beliefs, Nidra welcomes you. While its roots are in Eastern culture, it's wholly accessible for all people. A good teacher would not force their personal beliefs down your throat. Nidra typically shares rather generalized anecdotes and philosophical concepts without going too deep into theology or anything of the sort.

Nidra doesn't fit in my religion ... Do you enjoy the practice? If so, you can likely make it work. When your teacher speaks of "Spirit" or "Source energy," could you replace their words with a term you understand? How might you further blend your religious beliefs with Nidra? Explore the similarities between your religion and Nidra. From your perspective, are they both rooted in love? In introspection? Emphasize the similarities, rather than the differences, between your faith and Nidra. You can create a personal practice specific to your needs and beliefs so that you can continue enjoying Nidra no matter what religion you practice.

I took a yoga class one time and I didn't enjoy it . . . Nidra is noticeably different from a typical yoga asana class, as it is more similar to savasana. No one watches you. You won't stare into a mirror for an hour. There are no poses to move throughout. You don't need to be "physically fit." You simply need a body, a mind, and breath. Nidra might be the *most simple*, yet transformative, yoga out there.

Group classes aren't for me . . . You can practice Nidra entirely on your own. As an introvert myself, I completely hear you on this one. Sometimes showing up to a packed studio is just not in the books. Practice in a space where you feel comfortable. Nidra recordings can easily be found on the internet, so hop onto the web and surf your way to a practice that works for you.

Getting to know your mind

In Patanjali's *Yoga Sutras*, yoga is defined as "annulling the ripples of the mind." What could this mean? The ripples of the mind are thoughts. To annul means to "declare invalid." Yoga asks those walking the path to acknowledge that their thoughts are invalid. I would not say that means to deny your entire perception, but rather to consider where your thoughts come from especially those that do not serve you. We perceive only a sliver of reality.

Through yoga, we are able to explore the inner depths and the roots of illusions and ripples. Yoga allows us to see ourselves beyond our thoughts—for we are not the endless ripples parading through our waking consciousness. To "annul the ripples of the mind" might mean we can transcend thought and accept that we are more than the stories we tell ourselves.

Dealing with Distractors

Finding a *perfectly* quiet space to practice Nidra is practically impossible. Big cities, playful children, beloved pets, nearby street noises, and all sorts of sounds flood our spaces. Be patient with your distractions. If a loved one encroaches on your space, accidentally or otherwise, take a moment and find a breath. Honor the ways of this practice. Now might be a time to practice both non-reaction and non-attachment. Pause prior to speaking ill to anyone. Release yourself from personal expectations of your practice.

Personally, I have found it difficult to return to my interrupted practice if I react harshly or out of frustration. I disrupted myself more than the other interruption. My own actions were more detrimental than other factors. And it is important for me to remember that I have more control over myself than anything or anyone else. So take control for a moment, even if you are deep in your practice of stillness and surrender.

Hold yourself accountable for showing up for your practice in an unexpected way. By maintaining peace beyond your practice, you can face the distraction, communicate respectfully and return to your space without jarring yourself.

Allowing distractions can be the best option at times. If your mind feels especially loud and rowdy one day, ride the waves. Let them go wild for a bit. Go through your usual rituals and techniques, but if they simply are *not* doing the trick, then let your mind be as it wishes. Not every practice will be "perfect" and transformative. If it were, then a lot more folks would be enlightened by now.

Honor Your Unfurling

Bearing witness to all you are, even just bits and pieces at a time takes its toll. The inner realms of self are not filled with rainbows and butterflies. While the ultimate "end" of this path can be incredibly light and joyous, part of the path requires you to explore darkness and shadow. After some of your practices, you might feel as if a dark shadow followed you out of your space. From personal experience, this lingering heaviness is occasionally appropriate and will shed shortly thereafter.

Think of it this way: You are equal parts light, dark, and shadow. When "light" follows you beyond a practice space, do you attempt to shake it off? Or do you lean in and explore it, steep yourself in its bliss? In the hopes of better getting to know yourself, beyond the ego, encourage you to lean into the dark as well. Listen to its whispers. Allow it to linger awhile, as you would do for the light. Honor its ways as it is as much a part of you as your light. Light is cherished in modern society, but darkness can also bring about transformation and healing.

Darkness is not necessarily "bad," nor is light entirely "good.'" Release the labels we place upon the words used to describe our energy and essence. We are incredibly complex energetic beings, and categorizing different essences as "good" or "bad" will not aid in your progression toward awareness and enlightenment.

Comfort is key, especially when you are first coming to understand your body and how it moves in and out of a meditative state. Props are your friend and can offer you support as needed. Despite what most of us *want* to believe, our human bodies are incredibly fragile. Honor such fragility. Be *humbled* by your delicacy.

Support your physical vessel with props and blankets as needed. Oftentimes, students' egos take a blow when they see themselves in need of a prop, but the person beside them does not. Release your ego. On any other day, your fellow students might use *plenty* of props, and they simply are not in need of them on this one day. Allow your practice to be entirely yours. Shed any focus placed upon others.

Which props are best? The following are most yogis' go-tos:
- Bolster—can support the spine, head, and neck
- Meditation cushion—aid in lengthening your spine in a seated position
- Blanket—one which can be easily folded into different sizes
- Blocks—ideal for support, can be used for knees, shoulders, head, or neck

Setting Stones

In a bit, I will ramble on about how this path is directionless. For those new to cultivating intuition, it might be necessary to pave your way with a few intentionally placed "stepping stones." Learning to listen to your intuition and inner guides takes time. And, it might include a few missteps. Intuition arises differently in all of us. For some, they feel it bubble up in their mind—a thought that is as clear as a bluebird day. Others might find their intuition to be most potent in their center—their gut feelings *really* have some wise words and nudges. Explore where your intuition thrives and find practices that cultivate the energy and power of that space.

The stones you might set into place relate to maintaining consistency in your practice and creating a habit that lasts. You can find a 21-day guide on exploring and sticking to your Nidra practice at the back of the book, including stepping stones like:

- Getting to know your breath and the benefits of release, regulation, and direction
- Fleshing out the meaning of your Sankalpa and its direct purpose, relation to you and specifics
- Creatively curating your practice specific to you, your needs, and your present state of being on a given day
- Easing in and out of your practice, especially if you are practicing Nidra solo without a teacher to vocally guide you through the transitions of internalization and externalization
- Harmonizing the many layers within yourself to that of your practice and its depths

Non-Attachment

With these stepping stones set in place to give you an outline as you begin to forge ahead you might find yourself *incredibly* attached to the results. Enter, *non-attachment*. You might have heard of attachment before. Perhaps you are familiar with the well-known and widely shared wisdom from the Noble Truths of Zen Buddhism. The Second Noble Truth states, "the origin of suffering is attachment."

What exactly is *attachment*, though? To some, attachment bears a negative connotation and could be likened to a sort of frowned upon "clingy-ness." While the aggressively negative connotation should be shed (is that not a form of attachment?), the connection to "clinging" stands close to what attachment is all about.

Attachment is a sort of grasping for a certain result, experience, person, state of being, or desire. You might be attached to something physical. Humans tend to cling to material items as a means of fulfillment.

In yogic traditions, attachment is seen as a negative as it detracts from an individual's inner journey and spiritual fulfillment. The craving of material goods, wealth, or lusting of another is thought to pave the way to suffering rather than enlightenment. From a slightly shifted perspective, attachment connects to an aversion to something. You can be attached to what you *do not* desire to have or experience.

Regarding your personal practice, releasing attachment and approaching your path without expectation is wildly beneficial. Simply trusting in yourself, Spirit energy, and your practice to unfurl as they will is a beautiful way to walk forward. Attachment slows. Attachment might steer you into a vat of quicksand. The murky depths of walking within are lightened when you have no expectations. You walk ahead without picturing what enlightenment might be and when it will arrive. Carrying ideals and high expectations of a picturesque or quick journey will only slow your walk, giving the murky depths time to churn and become muddy.

Explore your attachments. *Greet* them. Say, "*Hello*, desire for fast results" and acknowledge the craving of a relationship that does not aid in growth—thoughts of where you *want* to be in a year from now in your practice.

Ask yourself and your attachments: What expectations are you carrying with you? Are they weighing you down, slowing your roll? How can you release them? How can you move forward with *nothing* in mind regarding what might come your way or where your path might lead?

These might sound like daunting questions, but they're entirely worth rumination. A thousand times over, you might return to one attachment or another and ask it to bid you farewell. Attachments cling too. They run deep and cutting their visible blossoms does not always do the trick. Only uprooting the attachment entirely will banish it. Such uprooting takes time, as does the entirety of this path.

In the *Bhagavad Gita*, a Sanskrit text, yoga is defined as "the discipline which severs the connection with that which causes suffering." Let's explore this quote a bit.

Suffering links to attachment and desires. Yoga asks students to stray away from the connection to the material world and its ways of envy, lust, and greed. In straying away, threads are cut. Yogis grow to become all the more capable of standing entirely fulfilled within themselves. The need for outside gain and grasping for "more" dissipates. As in all things, of course, attachment and the severing of this connection comes and goes. It bears a cyclical nature. Over time, with consistency and discipline, you might find yourself retreating further and further away, until one day, the thread snaps for good.

The Way of Simplicity

Now, after all that talk about additions to your practice, I'll offer an alternative, perhaps a bit more minimalist type of practice. Simplicity is equally as blissful in many ways. The nature of simplicity, light, soft, and filled with ease, can allow your Nidra practice to unfold all on its own.

In the world of yoga, where so many options presently exist and more are made available every year, less can be more. If you don't have access to fancy props, a pillow or your favorite blanket will do. Books can replace cork blocks. Any flooring with a decent amount of grip can carry you just as well as a yoga mat.

Simplifying your practice can aid in its transformation. If you feel stuck in your path, overwhelmed with the options presented before you, or unsure which route is "best" for you, cut back on what you are consuming. Step back from the marketing ploys and call outs. Retreat to your heart space, where light, dark, and shadow dance, and move from there. Practice with less. Practice in solitude. Turn off the lights, drop your eyes shut, and gaze within. To practice Nidra, all you really need is yourself.

Finding a Rhythm

Diligence, or "tapas," requires an awareness of your personal rhythms. At what point in the day do you find yourself craving a moment to recharge? Prior to that moment, what events drained your energy? Through the careful observation of your present routines, you can find the best times and ways to weave Nidra into your days.

For instance, you might find yourself feeling zapped around 3 p.m. Leading up to that, you might have had an incredibly full day. Would it benefit you to practice Nidra around 3 p.m., or could you find sometime earlier in the day before the exhaustion hits? You might feel more motivated to practice Nidra once you already feel exhausted, but it could be beneficial to beat your exhaustion to the punch. Practicing Nidra while you are more alert will likely lessen your chances of falling asleep or drifting away from your present mind and breath.

Thanks to the influence of the seasons, certain weeks of the year might urge you to practice more than usual. During summertime, when the sun's beams push individuals to play more than rest, you might feel *less* motivated to practice Nidra, despite the increased benefits during this time. As the weather cools, autumn offers especially cozy days that might have you moving deeper into your practice.

Come winter, the peak time for curling up within and finding rest, you might benefit from a more uplifting Nidra practice. If you practice on your own, you can tweak your practice to include more energizing visuals and breath. If you attend Nidra classes guided by a teacher, you could ask your teacher to incorporate elements that are more invigorating.

Nidra as "Self-Care"

If you're finding it difficult to make time for your practice, consider your perspective. How are you viewing Nidra? Is it a practice you turn to in hopes of awakening within? Are you returning time and time again without growing as you thought you would? Do you drag your feet when finding your way to your practice?

Frame Nidra within the recently popularized "self-care" realm of wellness. While caring for yourself has always been a well-known "must," only recently did self-care routines become something worth building, properly maintaining, and sharing with others. Place Nidra within your self-care rituals. If you use a face mask once per week, find similar time for Nidra. Prioritize Nidra as a must rather than a "maybe."

In a consumerist culture such as ours in the Western world, we are faced with *so* much marketing geared toward self-care and wellness. The wellness industry has begun to capitalize on Eastern philosophies to the point where some offerings are inauthentic. By practicing Nidra, you can still dabble in self-care and enhance your wellness while honoring its ancient roots. It's a practice directly related to you and experienced almost entirely within. There's no exploitation or obnoxious marketing scheme involved—it's a minimal practice that offers maximum results in overall well-being.

Finding Teachers

If I have learned anything in my years of studying yoga and Eastern philosophy, it's this: *Teachers come as you are ready for them*. Following up on that, teachers also *leave* (or, you choose to part ways with their teachings) when such a time comes.

You might absolutely adore a teacher's style, voice, or energy for months, years, decades. If one day comes and you suddenly sense you are distancing yourself from them, check in with this experience. Shifting from teacher to teacher, or spending some time without a consistent and clear teacher, can be helpful. At the end of this path, you might realize you are your own greatest teacher. All you need and crave dances within your being. You need only explore within, through Nidra and whichever other practices call you, and dig up the depths of the self. Sometimes a teacher aids in such digging. At other phases in your life, you might be the only one who can guide your inner gaze and fuel the movement of shoveling through your murky depths.

From a teacher's perspective, I can tell you I wholeheartedly understand all aspects of building a relationship and distancing. I have experienced this process myself, as a student moving away from one teacher and arriving at another. As I teacher, I have witnessed the very same in my students wandering away from my classes and teachings. Not once have I been offended. These paths are often intertwined with one another, then veer off in another way. Teachers come and go, as in all things, and will gladly welcome you back if you ever wish to return. We understand that you are your greatest guide, for only you know your body, spirit, and intuition on an intimate level.

Trust your intuition, those "pings" and "dings" in your mind's eye or your gut, to direct you. Allow the depths of self to carry you to and from teachers. Directions are complex on the path you walk. One might even say it's a directionless path, and that's the magic of its ways.

A Need For Nidra

I touched on this earlier, but our modern Westernized society craves Nidra without even fully realizing it as the Yin-like aspects of rest balance the heightened and overwhelming nature of our Yang-tendencies, such as working overtime. If you have any doubts, I'll detail a few major shifts in society that express our need for yoga Nidra's soothing ways.

- Screen time over quality time—Not long ago, I spent an entire week without my phone. Beforehand, I genuinely felt stressed about going so long without my tiny, handheld computer. That week, though, I felt more free and connected than I had in years. While they do offer us a lot of 'pros,' the 'cons' of smartphones run rampant. Walking down the street, you are more likely than ever to bump into someone staring down at their phone rather than watching where they were going. The introspection experienced in Nidra offers a moment of reflection we cannot receive from staring into a phone or laptop screen. Of course individuals love Nidra. True quiet time and inner wandering are seldom found in the heads down, internet-crazed Western world.

- Immediacy over patience—Running along a similar vein, the frenzy of social media and online shopping, among other digital activities, now places the sensation of immediacy at the top of society's priority list. Society, having grown accustomed to immediate results, lives by the thinking pattern: "If it won't ship in two days, then that's a major inconvenience." Something is posted online and could go viral, immediately changing someone's life. "Likes" on Instagram offer immediate validation. How fleeting is this immediate arrival of satisfaction and digital "abundance"? Results from Nidra don't always arrive with the same immediacy. Yet students return time and time again, as they come to embrace patience and continue to cultivate their practice. I have seen students who expect miracles from a yoga practice or meditation. Such immediacy is a rarity while walking this path, as hardly any spiritual or mental practice will offer the same quick results of the digital age. Nonetheless, students trek on, and often come to see how impatient society has become.

- Burnout rather than a steady flow. Imagine if the sun shone down on the entire Earth endlessly. The moon never rose into the skyline granting us a lunar guide toward darkness, sleep, and inner realms. For one, we would all be incredibly hot. The extra daylight would keep folks going, going, going just as many wish to continue. Of course, in Northern countries, this is the case. Notice, though, how they handle such endless daylight hours? They adjust and learn to "shut off" at a reasonable hour. In many ways, society's tendency to embrace spaces and habits relating to "never sleep" shows how out of rhythm we are. While we might find a way to grab some sleep, big cities, our smartphones, and a misconstrued notion that one *must* keep working often leads to detrimental burnout.

  Overworked and underslept, a functional society cannot continue in this way and expect all to be well. Nidra offers the nighttime element of lunar, feminine flow. Its growing popularity shows that it is needed in order to balance our incredibly Yang societal tendencies. Burnout is a closed door, whereas a steady ebb and flow of productivity levels and energy can continue on for an indefinite amount of time.

Nidra allows you to step away from your phone, gaze within, and slow down. If you practice in a community space, you can connect with others who are doing the same. Nidra has the power to massively shift and heal our world so that it might rest in balance.

Honoring vs. Appropriating Culture

When studying Eastern philosophy and culture, it's incredibly important to honor all you find especially if you are benefiting from the culture in some way. Take the time to understand the roots of the yoga practice. Get to know the controversies that have bubbled up over the years regarding the Westernization of Eastern concepts.

Be humbled by yourself at times. There is no harm in owning the fact that you might have made some disrespectful decisions in the past when you were unaware. Stepping up and acknowledging your own mistakes shows growth and encourages others in the yoga community to do the same.

When practicing, studying, or teaching yoga, you can either honor the culture or appropriate it. If yoga is not your culture, meaning you are not from the regions and religions which brought it into being, then become critically aware of how you go about engaging in the practice.

To honor the culture, participate in its practices without stealing ideas and making them your own in a disrespectful manner. Understand the symbols, words, and chants and use them properly and with respect. Study Sanskrit and learn to pronounce the words correctly. If you can pronounce the words correctly, use them often in your classes.

What does appropriation look like? It exists in varying ways. In one form, it is seen when a privileged person takes something from another culture and benefits from it in a way a person from the original culture would be unable to benefit. Teaching a yoga class with only yoga asana and no regard for philosophy, history, and culture can lean into an appropriative realm.

If an individual from the originating culture or community approaches you and shares concerns regarding your words or actions, remain open. Hear their words. They mean no harm, they simply wish to show you how you are stepping on the toes of their culture. If they ask you to make a change, be willing to shift your words or actions. Perhaps you mispronounced a word and they corrected you. Thank them for taking the time to tell you; they surely did not have to do that. It should have been your responsibility to know better.

In the realm of Nidra, it's important to honor the history and know the philosophy system in which it's based. If you choose to share or repeat Sanskrit mantras, be especially sure to pronounce them properly and know their meaning.

Cultivating a Home Nidra Practice

Comfort is a must. Prioritize coziness in your set-up, especially as you are beginning your practice. Maintain some semblance of comfort throughout your practice as it expands. Creating a sacred space within your home is a beautiful way to honor the practice. Plus, if the ambiance is right, you might be more inclined to tuck within the space and practice.

To curate a soothing and warm space, you might simply toss some soft pillows on the floor, light a candle, and call it a day. Simplicity is key, but don't be wary of abundance. Decorate your space as much or as little as you like. Pillows, bolsters, blankets, blocks, eye masks, and weighted blankets can amp up your practice.

With weighted blankets and eye masks shutting out any light, your time in Nidra can be more intense. Weighted blankets further aid in shifting you into your Parasympathetic Nervous System. They also tend to make you feel as if you are floating even more so than usual during a meditative state. If that sounds more unsettling than soothing, skip the weighted blanket. It is certainly not for everyone.

In your space, you might create an altar of sorts. By creating a clear, carefully cultivated space dedicated to your practice, you now have a physical reminder of that practice. It can call to you when you glance at it as you are rushing out the door in the morning. As you shut the door behind you, you might think, *Oh, yeah, I should spend some time in Nidra later today.* Your altar can feature anything near and dear to you. Anything that has come to you because of your practice, or perhaps some beauty that guided you to your practice in the first place. Your space reflects you and your inner world—allow it to shift accordingly.

Personally, I like to decorate my altar with seasonal influences. During springtime, I fill my space with florals and soft colors, perhaps some fresh flowers. Come summer, a season of abundance, I brighten the colors and invite in more of the season's earthly bounty. Candles, trinkets, seashells, incense, and gifts almost always find themselves featured on my altar. Winding into fall, my altar quiets a bit, shedding some of its layers with the season. Earth tones and autumn touches, such as gourds, dried oranges, and pumpkins, fill my space. A last, with winter, my altar features snow-inspired details, with light linens and white candles taking over.

Additional Sequencing Methods

At times, a Nidra practice might extend beyond the usual eight phases. Depending upon your teacher and guides, Nidra might sound different or be shared in a new form. Remain open to the varying methods and philosophies. You never know which might resonate with you. And it doesn't hurt to pick up some pieces of one method then bring it into another aspect of your practice.

One addition might be the recognition of the six stages of relaxation that unfold in correspondence with the *koshas* and Atma. For clarity, I'll detail the koshas for you before we get into the stages and their essences. The koshas are the five layers of being within all of us. That's right, we all have *five bodies*. The "outer" bodies are heartier than the "inner" layers. The inner koshas exist in a finer way than the outer. Originally, the koshas were detailed in the *Taittiriya Upanishad*, a Vedic-era Sanskrit text. The text wrote that "human beings consist of a material body built from the food they eat. Those who care for this body are nourished by the universe itself." Further along, it's shared that "inside this is another body made of life energy" and "within the vital force is yet another body, this one made of thought energy." It keeps going, detailing the following layers.

The innermost body, which I speak to explicitly below, "is yet a subtler body, composed of pure joy" and "it is experienced as happiness, delight, and bliss." To visualize the koshas, you can imagine them as sheaths over your body, or a Russian doll, where each piece fits perfectly within another. Ancient Indian yogis curated specific practices with the intent to hone in on each kosha and strengthen its life force.

Back to the relaxation progression featured in Nidra—the stages, following the *koshas*, are as follows:

1. Physical—*annamaya kosha*—"Maya" means "made of." "Anna" means "food." This is the physical body you likely know fairly well by now. It requires sustenance and nourishment through food and movement.

2. Energetic, Vital Energy Sheath—*pranamaya kosha*—In yoga, pranayama consists of practices of becoming aware, regulating, controlling, and shifting your breath. Without the proper functioning of your *pranamaya kosha*, fueling your energy, vitality shrinks.

Through yoga, you can become increasingly aware of all that goes into holding your body together. It's no small feat, that's for sure. This physical kosha connects and rules over your human processes keeping your body going. Your breathing, digestion, and blood circulation are included in this realm. Your life force, known as *prana* in yoga, vibrates here. Breath awareness in Nidra can grant you access to your *prana maya kosha*.

Often our energetic communication with events and people beyond ourselves occurs through this layer of being. Notice how you react, in breath and personal energy, when in the presence of someone incredibly sad or devastated. You likely "pick up" on their energy in some way, and such empathy might be due to this kosha's essence.

3. Mental—*manomaya kosha*—"Manomaya" means "body made of thought processes." While Western folks tend to liken thought to the brain and the brain alone, yoga considers the nervous system's role in things. Many yogis think the *mano maya kosha* might step in and play a role in the widespread communication of needs and demands through mind and body.

   Within the *manomaya kosha*, samskaras exist, energetic DNA can be grooved into your being without your conscious awareness. While meandering through the energetics of the *mano maya kosha*, you might be able to tap into these grooves and their patterns more than usual. We mentioned the grooves earlier—they show up as habitual behaviors and thought patterns which no longer benefit you. This stage is when the *samskaras* shift these deeply ingrained behaviors and thoughts, encouraging them to dissipate.

4. Intuitive, Wisdom/Awareness Body—*vijnanamaya kosha*—Diving deeper into inner worlds, the *vijnana maya kosha* contains ancient wisdom and knowledge. Intuition thrives in this layer. Insight and the call to create following a meditative or spiritual practice comes about from within these realms. Even while writing or creating in a fluid, deeply ritualistic manner, you channel the energy of the *vijnana maya kosha* without fully realizing it.

5. Joy, Bliss Body—*anandamaya kosha*—Lastly, the *ananda maya kosha* hides furthest within our bodies. It's felt as the innate knowledge that life is worthwhile and to contain to live is "good." This sheath tells you *you are born to experience the pure, unstoppable bliss of being*. A natural ecstasy pulsates through the *ananda maya kosha*. Mantra, meditation, and prayer (of any sort) digs you into the essence of the bliss body. When you feel overwhelming joy, pure ecstasy, and unexplainable happiness, you have tapped into your bliss body.

6. Atma awareness—Shifting away from koshas, the sixth stage presented here is *Atma*. Atma connects rather simply to the concept of "I." The "I" you speak of when you express needs, wants, desires, and feelings is surface-level. The "I" of Atma knows its vastness and divinity. Through the shedding of conscious thought and dissipation of ego, one can acknowledge and accept their Atma—knowledge of their natural state is one of pure consciousness. Such awareness brings about joy and liveliness unlike any other.

Awareness of these six stages requires a bit more practice than the usual Nidra session might offer. It can take years to come to know and feel into the koshas, so grant yourself patience in coming to know their ways within yourself. You might experience them in a fleeting moment, such as a blissful sensation on a summer's day with loved ones in a sacred setting, and have a sense of *ananda maya* pulling you inward.

Additional Insight: Chidakash and Hridayakasha

Following the visualization often offered in Nidra, you will likely come to rest in a space of pure introspection. This inner realm is called *Chidakash*, which roughly translates to "the space of mental consciousness." You might physically feel this space pulsating just inside your forehead, perhaps near your third eye chakra.

Another space, known as *Hridayakasha*, thrives in the heart space consciousness. Most often, *Hridayakash* resonates in the center of a person's chest. Both realms of energy, *Chidakash* and *Hridayakash*, offer space for inward exploration after a repetition of a mantra. In the case of Nidra, they follow the repetition of your Sankalpa for the second time.

While resting in these spaces, you take the seat of the non-judging witness once more. You allow yourself, your ways, your truth to unfurl in front of your "eyes" or "inner gaze." No reactions are necessary. As if you are watching a theatre production, you do not react or interact. You witness all you are but you are not involved in "all you are."

Ultimately, you are carried to this point of *Chidakasha* and *Hridayakash* through all the phases of Nidra leading up to the pure space dedicated to introspection. It's the final stage prior to externalization—when you return to the outer experiences of perceived reality. Within a "pure" experience of *Chidakasha* and *Hridayakash*, no manipulation, falsified perception or energetic shifts are possible or allowed. The raw truth of who you are, how you are, and why you are might be shown to you. Oftentimes, these realities are incredibly difficult to swallow. On the surface level, we take in only mirrored visions of ourselves—through our interactions with one another, channeled creativity, spoken words, attachment to thoughts, literal glass reflections. So to witness our raw "self" can be jarring to some but, when accepted, is immensely soothing. Such acceptance of self shown to you without ego and body is known as *Samadhi*, which we touched on a few chapters ago.

Tracking Your Journey

Journaling adds a beautiful bit of record-keeping to your practice. Honoring your progress is an often-forgotten aspect. Prior to glancing back at your steps to where you stand presently, you might be entirely oblivious to the progress you have made thus far.

Journal entries require only as much effort as you wish to expel. One day, you might write ten pages and experience a massive brain dump. The next, you can only write a word or two before you feel uninterested. This is another example of the ebbs and flows of your path and practice.

At times when you feel stagnant, I encourage you to think back on where you were a year ago, a week ago, or yesterday. Our beings and minds change subtly by the minute and vastly over great stretches of time. We remain primarily unaware of these shifts. Through journaling, you can track your experiences and witness your transformation in a more grounded sense than simply *feeling* as if you might have grown a bit. You *have* grown! Honor that and be humbled by your own knowledge and greatness.

Stimulating Creativity

Building a bridge between your conscious mind, which produces tangible art and writing, and your unconscious, linked to the Divine more clearly, can allow for your creative process to transcend its present ways. If you have felt "stuck" creatively, Nidra can allow your mind to expand. Over time, achieving a heightened state of consciousness repeatedly can truly transform your art and the creative process. Looking at the basic concept of "relaxation" as soothing yourself to a point where your mind can be quiet, allows for terrific thoughts to come to the surface.

When you think about the well-known idea of "shower thoughts"—where individuals claim they have simply *the best* thoughts in the shower—what is happening? They are calm. They aren't racing about with a million thoughts at any given moment. *Of course,* you have ideas in the shower when you are more present than you might be when going about your errands and chipping away at your to-do list. The shower grants most people a moment of rest in-between stressors. It is a peaceful space, even if you only have a moment to rinse off. Imagine how many "shower thoughts" you could have in an entire hour practice of Nidra? You could write a book with all the wisdom coming from the quiet corners of your mind!

Expanding Your Yoga

In addition to your Nidra practice, you can explore other styles of meditation and yoga. Personally, I have found a melding of beliefs and rituals to be beneficial in cultivating a sustainable environment for sadhana and my personal growth. Plus, the fun of learning remains steady as I get to explore the many ancient words and ways of numerous cultures, philosophy systems, and traditional healing methods.

Outside of Nidra, where do you feel yourself called to explore? Does Yin Yoga and some of its methods call you? Yin Yoga offers a moving meditation of sorts. Each yin shape carries a different energy and moves your life force—prana—in a certain direction. One shape might ground you, and the next uplifts you. Yin Yoga aims to bring students into a balance while still allowing them to wander deeply within. Sounds familiar, right? A Yin Yoga class with a bit of Nidra offered at the end is not uncommon. Many Yin students and teachers dabble in Nidra, and vice versa. The subtle movements offered in Yin, with each shape acting as a container of meditation, might be a refreshing switch from total stillness. Sometimes consistent practices can lose their potency if we remain stagnant in our desire to learn and study yoga.

Other additions might include a form of sound therapy, such as a gong bath or Tibetan singing bowl. Sound therapy seems to benefit individuals seeking healing on an energetic level. Similar to Nidra, the musical notes and soundwaves connect to a healing space below the surface of your skin. Tensions can be released and old patterns moved through, all thanks to the gong or singing bowls. The sound waves wash over you and cleanse your energy field. You might find it beneficial to find a class offering sound therapy along with Nidra, or you can find sound therapy outside of Nidra. It can stand alone as a complementary healing method and further aid in the progression of your path.

As you grow to better understand Yoga Nidra, you might be able to offer it to yourself in a natural way. Once you come to know the pattern seen in rotating your consciousness from one body part to another, you might instinctually move through the rhythm in your own time. I have had students in my classes practice Reiki on themselves while in Savasana, and I fully support such a practice. For clarity, Reiki is a hands-on energetic practice. With the knowledge of specific energy centers and proper energetic alignment, a Reiki practitioner can bring themselves into balance simply by placing their hands on parts of their body and infusing the space with mental "pushes." Reiki or otherwise, you know best, and if you need some Nidra in your Savasana but it is not being shared by the teacher, give yourself that gift.

Beyond Nidra and Yin Yoga, you can explore other meditation methods. Nidra might not be accessible at all hours for you, and if you are feeling exhausted or stressed while commuting to work, another mindfulness technique could help. What other techniques could you carry with you in the moments when the depths of Nidra are unavailable but you need a pick-me-up? An alternative way to look at this is to think about how you can *simplify* Nidra so that it can act as an on-the-go tool. Can you carry your Sankalpa with you beyond your practice? Are you able to maintain an awareness of your breath when faced with conflict? Can you find the pause, the slow, the patient ways of Nidra throughout the hours off your mat?

Nidra Cheat Sheet

As we wind down in these final few pages, I would like to offer you a "Nidra Cheat Sheet." A wide amount of knowledge and concepts have filled these pages. I hope you are looking forward to continuing the exploration of your Nidra practice. Below I'll detail a few key points and concepts you can focus on beyond your actual practice. If you choose, you can continue to pursue the textual and philosophical realms of your Nidra practice, and allow it to transform your path in addition to the actual yoga Nidra.

- Prana—Your breath and life force. Dancing through you in all your days, how can you remain aware? Once, I read a spiritual text that encouraged students to mind their breath while sitting at a red light. No matter how late you are to whatever appointment, can you pause and be present in the beauty of your breath? The light will change when it is ready—you have absolutely zero control. Your breath, though? You have the power to shift that at any given moment, and you know how healing that is despite your inability to process such pranic shifts in flow.

- Sacred texts—Reading brings about peace too. Same with audiobooks, as a matter of fact! If you have absolutely loved the mentions of ancient texts and scriptures, you can hop over to the nearest bookshop and grab a copy. Dig the books apart and eat them up. Consume the wisdom in a tangible, academic manner. It's a way to honor these ancient cultures and find growth all at once.

- Sankalpa—Your Sankalpa extends so far beyond your practice and your mat, whether you realize it or not. How can you continue to move with your Sankalpas beyond your space and allow them to transform you? Try writing yours down in a journal or on a sticky note. Dog-ear the page or place the note somewhere you can see it every day.

- The Witness—Taking the seat of the witness to all you are, benefits you in nearly every moment. It grants you greater presence and brings a gentle interaction to your approach to inner "self" vs. outer "self." Remain aware of the witness and how they are always there—watching without judgment or direct thought as your days unfurl.

- Listen to intuition—Honor the moments where you quite simply *crave* a moment of peace. You might grow more reliant on your practice than you once thought possible. If you have missed a few days of practice, or could not find a Nidra class while out of town, take the time to cultivate this need for quiet and introspection.

- Reflection—There are mirrors within and beyond you. See them and allow yourself to *be seen*. Earlier on, in the first chapter, we considered the purpose of Nidra. After all this, you might come to see that Nidra acts as a transportation system within so that you might see all that you already are. Through Nidra, you gain access to halls, walls and doorways within your inner landscape that were once locked and shut. Nidra gives you the most beautiful, everlasting bounty—inner reflection.

Cultivating a vision all your own

As you go along, you will understand your preferences and needs, even as they shift and transform. You hold the power in your practice. Choose the teachers you enjoy—perhaps due to their lovely, melodic voice, or because of their ability to keep you awake with their presence. Find the props which work with your body, and grant yourself the time to place them where they need to rest.

The cultivation of your practice comes with time, and it started the moment you first stepped *toward* this path and practice. Tune in to what works for you and what doesn't. You are worthy of a sublime and beneficial practice. Step into your worthiness and show up consistently as your best self, however that looks on any given day. Eventually, your practice can become a beautiful creation, entirely your own.

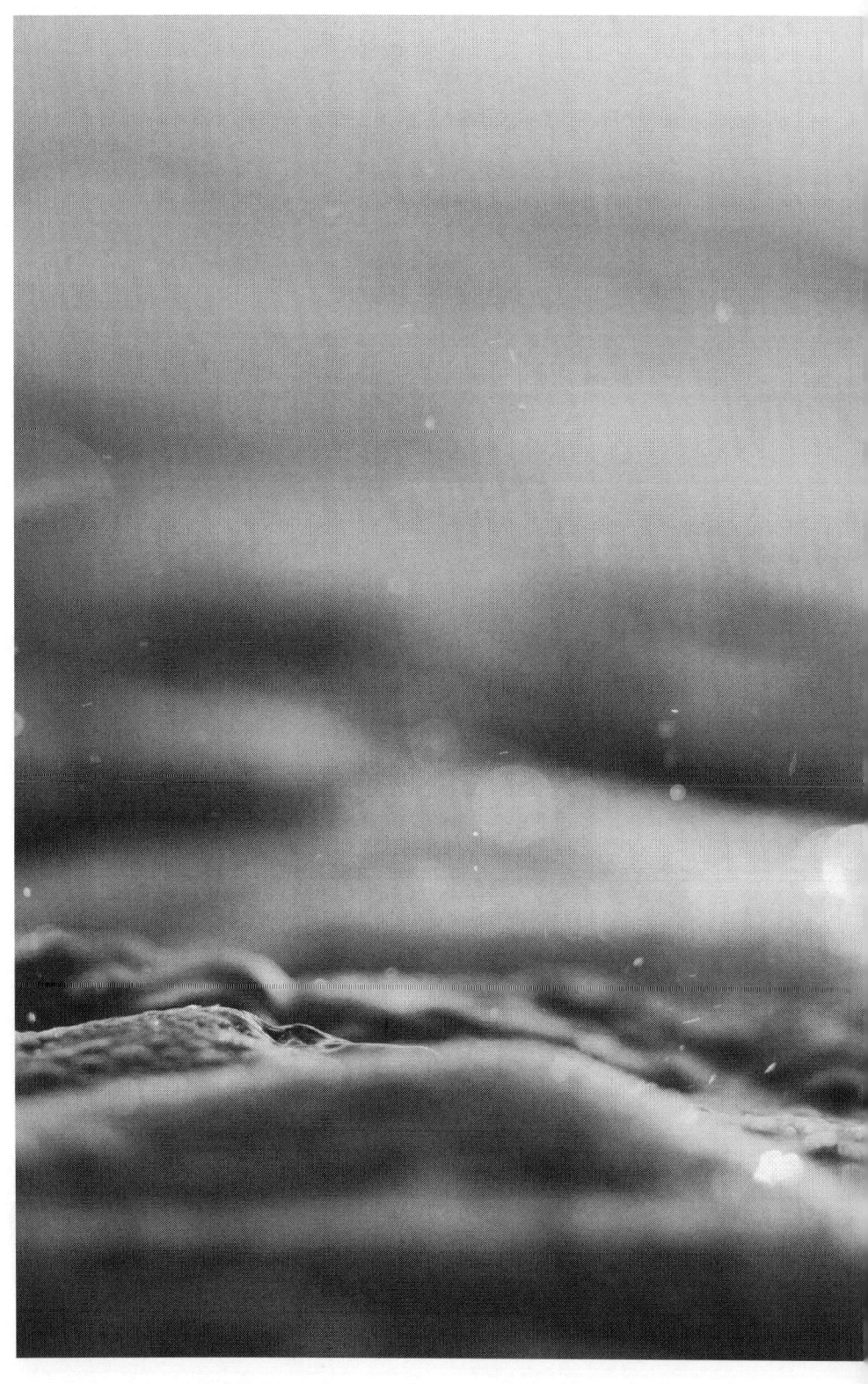

Chapter 8: 21-Day Challenge

Showing up for yourself

Over the course of the next three weeks, I'm asking you to show up for yourself as best as you can. Each day might look different. One day, you might fall into the rhythms of Nidra with minimal effort. Another, you might shy away from your practice space, or run away *quickly* in the other direction.

Showing up, as you might have heard from *a million* other yoga teachers, is the most difficult part, hands down. And there is a reason so many teachers share this bit of wisdom: It's true for so many of us. We all have days where getting our practice in feels like pulling teeth. How you feel after your practice, though, makes the teeth-pulling entirely worthwhile. Show up, because you *know* you deserve the bliss, the deepened awareness, and the beauty of Nidra.

Build a habit through these daily journal prompts, questions, and notes meant to guide you deeper into your personal practice. Take what serves you, leave the rest.

To kick things off, you'll be encouraged to grow more familiar with the cyclical, spiraling ways of your mind. Sending you love, blessings, and ease as you wander this 21-day path of Nidra.

Cycle 1: Getting to know the cyclical nature of your mind

Day 1: Here we are, building a beautiful consistency in your practice, all for you and your Spirit. Day by day, I'll guide you through some specific things to focus on in order to better grow and come to *witness* your practice. Today, we'll begin by exploring the wandering tendencies of the human brain and I'll offer you some questions on *how* you react to such wanders.

Before you begin, take note of how you are feeling *now* and check in with yourself after. I'll ask you to do this every day, so get ready for *a lot* of introspective moments.

At present, before my practice, I am feeling/experiencing:

Focus: During today's practice, count how many times your mind wanders prominently away from the presence, your breath, your Sankalpa.

After my practice, I am feeling/experiencing:

Introspection: How did you react to the wandering occurrences? Did your reaction serve you?
How might you react, or *not* react, the next time something disruptive occurs during your Nidra practice?

Day 2:

At present, before my practice, I am feeling/experiencing:

Focus: During today's practice, if/when your mind wanders, envision a thread, perhaps glistening silver or gold, wrapping itself around your "mind." The thread, with your breath and Spirit in control, gently tugs on your mind, drawing you back to the center.

After my practice, I am feeling/experiencing:

Introspection: Did the practice of "threading" aid in centering your mind today? What other ways might you focus your mind? What does "non-reaction" mean to you? Does "non-reaction" play out in other areas of your life, outside of your spiritual practices?

Day 3:

At present, before my practice, I am feeling/experiencing:

Focus: During today's practice, notice if any spirals or cycles of your mind feel familiar. Make a mental note of thoughts, patterns, phrases, or emotions that you might have experienced before.

After my practice, I am feeling/experiencing:

Introspection: Which thoughts or patterns were familiar to you? How do they continue to show up? When was the last time they showed up? Or an alternative question, how long have they been showing up in your mind? Are these thoughts and patterns serving you (i.e., aiding in your awakening and growth)? If so, how? If not, how might you release them? Are you prepared to release them from your mind and being?

Day 4:

At present, before my practice, I am feeling/experiencing:

Focus: Hone in on presence in its entirety. Practice simply today, allow for past lessons and realization to show up as they may.

After my practice, I am feeling/experiencing:

Introspection: How did today's practices and notes compare to Day 1? How would you like to feel by Day 11 next week? Day 21 in a couple of weeks? What can you do to continue to grow and arrive in those spaces?

Day 5:

At present, before my practice, I am feeling/experiencing:

Focus: During today's practice, to wrap up exploring the cyclical, remain fully present to the best of your ability. After your practice, we'll throw in a creative twist.

After my practice, I am feeling/experiencing:

Introspection: Today, rather than questioning in a cut and dry manner as we have on the days prior, I'll ask you to explore a more artistic route.
Draw a spiral on a piece of paper. Within your spiral, draw or write in the thoughts, patterns, feelings which arose during today's practice. If it helps, you can include some of the observa-

tions you gathered earlier this week. There's no right way to go about this, simply put pen to paper and let the cycles of your mind show themselves in a more tangible manner.

Hold onto this paper for now, and we will come back to it in a couple of weeks.

Cycle 2: Exploring your breath and present Sankalpa

Day 6:

A fresh start of sorts arrives with day 6. Today, attention and sadhana shift toward your breath and present Sankalpa. Over the next couple of days, you will be asked to explore the potency of your breath, its conversation with Divinity, and the foundations—the "why," of your present Sankalpa.

The same rhythm you settled into last week remains. Practice for a significant amount of time each day and jot down some thoughts, feelings, or rambles before you begin. Check back in with yourself after returning to the external world following your practice.

At present, before my practice, my breath is:
And, my focus is on:

Focus: During today's practice, count how many times your mind wanders prominently away from the presence, your breath, your Sankalpa. Count gently without expectation, reaction, or judgment as you go along. Our wandering minds are in our nature, and Nidra acts as a means to lessen such wandering, but might never fully "stop" this behavior of the mind.

After my practice, my breath is:
And, my focus is on:

Introspection: How did you react to the wandering occurrences? Did your reaction serve you?

How might you react, or *not* react, the next time something disruptive occurs during your Nidra practice?

Day 7:

At present, before my practice, my breath is:
And, my focus is on:

Focus: Observe your present state of being. Are you feeling rushed? For today's practice, emphasize your *exhales* to aid in release and slowing down. On the other hand, are you feeling a bit sleepier than usual? If so, lengthen your *inhales* to stir your mind and wake you up.

After my practice, my breath is:
And, my focus is on:

Introspection: Through the awareness, and some regulation, of your breath, what shifts occurred? What breathing pattern settled best in your practice today?

How might you bring these breathing patterns, awareness, and control methods into other realms of your life? How might you *remember* to weave such awareness and regulation into your daily routine and potential obstacles (such as sleepiness or heightened stress), in a subtle, but consistent, manner?

Day 8:

At present, before my practice, my breath is:
And, my focus is on:

Focus: Shifting away from your breath today, I'll ask you to explore your Sankalpa. What is your present focus, mantra, intention? Apply diligence to the repetition of your Sankalpa today. Envision it in all its layers. Place a color or two, or an entire rainbow, to your Sankalpa and allow it to *flood* your being. Your Sankalpa saturates all you are on a cellular level. Allow this to occur.

After my practice, my breath is:
And, my focus is on:

Introspection: Peruse the foundations and essences of your Sankalpa. How did it come to you? How long has this Sankalpa been a part of your practice? If your Sankalpa has been with you for quite some time, which is entirely subjective, is it still serving you? What did it mean to you upon first choosing it? Has its meaning, definition, or essence changed over time?

Day 9:

At present, before my practice, my breath is:
And, my focus is on:

Focus: Consider developing your Sankalpa a bit. Allow it to *guide* you today after having saturated your being a bit more potently in yesterday's practice. Ask your Sankalpa to carry you through its essence and purpose. As you wander within, Sankalpa takes the role of the guide today as you remain the witness. To be a witness means to observe all you are without judgment or expectation. You are seated in your mind's eye, seeing, though not directly interacting with, all that unfurls within.

After my practice, my breath is:
And, my focus is on:

Introspection: Write down your current Sankalpa. Explore every word. What does each word mean to you? Sometimes, with abstract words, such as "love," "joy," "success," and "positivity," we place others' definitions upon them more so than our own. We might not even be aware of this occurrence. Here's an example of how this might look:

An example Sankalpa: *I awaken my positive life force as I connect with others*

Word by word, here's how I would interpret the meaning of each word. The abstractions here are mainly *awaken—positive—life—force—connect*

I—For me, *I* represents all I am. My breath, my body, my spirit, my mind, my ego. So, I am aiming to awaken all I am, not just the *I* that relates readily to ego or conscious thought. Further, I often connect *I* to a more generalized sense of *"we"* as I believe in the shared collective consciousness. In invoking this *I* within the self, I sense that my inner work extends into the collective.

Awaken—To awaken is to stir the depths of my being. To wander the murky depths and let the ocean floor and its mysteries rise to the surface. To awaken is to find myself not only rising with the sun but rising at dusk, arriving firmly into my darkness. Awakening means, for me, to rise into a space where I can truly *see* all my layers, all my rooms within myself.

From there, continue on until you have fleshed out the more clear-cut meanings of every word and what they mean to you alone.

Day 10:
At present, before my practice, my breath is:
And, my focus is on:

Focus: Your focus remains on your Sankalpa today. This time, see if you can keep in mind the complexities, or simplicities, brought up through the word exploration exercise from yesterday. Keep your specific meanings for each word, every abstract, every *I* in your Sankalpa in mind as you allow it to saturate your being once more and guide you within.

After my practice, my breath is:
And, my focus is on:

Introspection: Did your Sankalpa guide you in any new directions today? Was your practice any different from the days prior? What shifts occurred, if any? No harm if today's practice remained the same as usual, more or less. That might mean your words were already fairly unique and specific.

Day 11:

At present, before my practice, my breath is:
And, my focus is on:

Focus: Notice the tense used in your Sankalpa. Do you say "I am" or "I will" in your repetition? No right or wrong answer, simply note which you are using. If you would like, shift into speaking with the present tense if you are using "I will" and vice versa if speaking in the present tense.

After my practice, my breath is:
And, my focus is on:

Introspection: Did shifting the tense of your Sankalpa shift your practice at all? Did you feel more present using one tense versus the other? Would you be inclined to keep one tense more than another in your affirmations? When might present tense serve you? When might future tense better serve you?

Cycle 3: Feeling into physical sensations and the experience of oppositions

Day 12:

Shifting focus, round two! For our first day of this cycle, we'll be honing in on the often-ethereal experience of sensation in Nidra. As yogis often lose "sense" of their physicality in Nidra, we'll take a creative route in exploring such sensations. Oftentimes, experiences in meditation and transcendence cannot be properly summed up in written words. This week, colored pencils, watercolors, a sketchbook, or some basic writing utensils will be beneficial.

At present, before my practice, my body feels:
And, overall, my emotions feel:

Focus: As you drop into your practice today, arrive with an open mind and spirit. Embrace the often ethereal, "airy," ways of Nidra. Be carried in the winds of your practice today. Draw in the practice of equanimity—non-judgment, non-reaction, non-labeling—and simply *be* in these winds.

After my practice, my body feels:
And, overall, my emotions feel:

> *Introspection:* Grab for some colored writing utensils or paints. Just two or three colors will do, even black and blue pens will do the trick. Find a blank piece of paper, or create your art on this very page, on these very words. *Paint, doodle, sketch, splash* your Nidra experience onto your paper today. Allow your breath to guide you. Allow your intuition to extend out through your hand into your materials. A creative brain dump, if you will, is your post-practice exercise for today.

Day 13:

At present, before my practice, my body feels:
And, overall, my emotions feel:

> *Focus:* Fall into an awareness of *opposition* today. Your main focus will be geared toward this state of your practice. If, and likely *when*, your mind wanders, draw it back toward the end of your practice as the experience of oppositions begins.

After my practice, my body feels:
And, overall, my emotions feel:

> *Introspection:* Which oppositions did you feel today? You can either *write* these out or return to a similar form of expression to yesterday's exercise. We'll circle back to this expression of opposites in tomorrow's practice.

Day 14:

At present, before my practice, my body feels:
And, overall, my emotions feel:

> *Focus:* Harmonization of opposition. Allow your experience of oppositions to meld together. Yesterday, in cultivating a greater awareness of opposites, you likely pushed them further apart. Today, encourage them, through breath and awareness of being, to dance together.

After my practice, my body feels:

And, overall, my emotions feel:

> *Introspection:* Having perhaps experienced a bit of harmony as oppositions arose within, express your experience on the same paper or page as yesterday's artistic expression. Paint, draw, write alongside or atop the work you shared yesterday. Explore how the two oppositions in and of themselves—harmony and polarity—melt into one another on paper.

Day 15:

At present, before my practice, my body feels:

And, overall, my emotions feel:

> *Focus:* Today, harmonize your body and mind. Grow your awareness of the dance between body, mind, breath, and Spirit. Hear how your breath dances in tune with the rhythmic guidance of your heart. Feel into the spaces where Spirit shines through the mind and its rambles subside. Come into a state of melodic flow. Allow the mind to be a low hum and Spirit to rise, rise, rise.

After my practice, my body feels:

And, overall, my emotions feel:

> *Introspection:* What rose up in your practice today? Through fluidity, where did you find yourself? How might you weave such fluidity into spaces and rituals, routines, or tasks outside of your direct Nidra practice?

Day 16:

At present, before my practice, my body feels:

And, overall, my emotions feel:

> *Focus:* Wrapping up our final day of this third cycle, today. With that, I'll ask you to find some movement prior to your Nidra practice today. Subtle or wild. In your arms, fingers, toes, neck, belly. Move as you feel called to. Linger in the spots where movement feels sticky. Marinate in the beauty of movement. Allow it to unfurl from the depths which you have been stirring.

After my practice, my body feels:
And, overall, my emotions feel:

Introspection: Having moved prior to entering your Nidra practice, did you experience a shift at all in comparison to other days? What did the movement stir up for you? How does stillness arrive in your body following movement? How did movement arise in the first place—was it welcomed, natural? Or, stagnant and timid? Witness the answers which might arise from these questions without judgment, always.

Cycle 4: Dropping in and rising out with ease, grace, and patience

Day 17:

As we close in this final fourth cycle, we will explore the processes of internalization and externalization. Rightfully so, being bookends, the two carry a lot of weight and have similarities. Moving in and out of the sacred Nidra state of being might be unpleasant. Or perhaps you struggle with arriving in such a state. Maybe both tend to be tricky for you! Either way, there are ways to better ease in and out of Nidra.

At present, before my practice, I am thinking about:
My mind, breath, and Spirit feel:

Focus: Shaking out your thoughts and wiggles *before* arriving fully to your Nidra practice. Movement comes along for the ride this week. Shake and shimmy about, imagine your thoughts, worries, to-dos floating up and out of your system. Let heaviness dissipate. Lighten up. Once your wiggles have all released, *then* shift into your practice properly.

After my practice, I am thinking about:
My mind, breath, and Spirit feel:

Introspection: Again, how did movement aid in the shift from your natural state to that of Nidra? Did your movement look different from yesterday to today? Did the differences come from an intuitive place or elsewhere? How might movement aid in other transitory spaces and ways in your daily life?

Day 18:

At present, before my practice, I am thinking about:
My mind, breath, and Spirit feel:

Focus: Arriving at our other bookend, today I will ask you to explore how you approach externalization. Leaving your practice, do the lights typically feel harsh and brutal? Well, *shift* that. Lower your gaze. Ask your teacher to dim the lights, if they can. Nidra asks us to release control, but outside elements remain under our control. Shut the blinds. Cover your eyes. Treat yourself gently as you submerge fully in darkness for today.

After my practice, I am thinking about:
My mind, breath, and Spirit feel:

Introspection: What does "darkness" mean to you? How does your darkness feel and appear to you? Can you tap into the relationship between your light, dark, and shadow essences?

Day 19:

At present, before my practice, I am thinking about:
My mind, breath, and Spirit feel:

Focus: Fragility. We humans love to run about, wild and free, which is beautiful. But until injury or something of the sort arises, we often forget to remember just how delicate we are. Such delicacy is humbling, yes. But it's also empowering when you are able to honor such fragility and move in a way that respects your bounds. After all, if you're this far along, your boundary-breaking is likely occurring in an intangible realm at this point. Move *slower than ever* in and out of any shapes you take throughout your day. Slow your walking pace. Let people pass. Slow is the way.

After my practice, I am thinking about:
My mind, breath, and Spirit feel:

Introspection: Did slowing down come easily to you, in your practice and otherwise? Do you have a sense of understanding your fragility? In what inner ways has Nidra cultivated strength within your being?

Day 20:
At present, before my practice, I am thinking about:
My mind, breath, and Spirit feel:

Focus: Approaching our bookends in a different way on our second to last day, today we will glance back to our earliest days. After all the varying "focuses" I've shared with you, which served you best? Which granted you some sort of realization or potent reaction (reactions happen, no matter how hard we try to not react)? Tap back into that space today. Go forward with no expectations despite recent experience.

After my practice, I am thinking about:
My mind, breath, and Spirit feel:

Introspection: Days, perhaps weeks, later—how does it serve you today? Would you explore this particular focus or exercise again, somewhere down the road?

Day 21:
At present, before my practice, I am thinking about:
My mind, breath, and Spirit feel:

Focus: At last, we (mainly, you!) have arrived. Arrive fully today. In harmony. In a quiet mind. In curiosity and gentle witnessing of all you are. Nourish yourself today however you feel called. Move before, or drop right in. Move after, or find space to remain in quiet stillness following your practice. Create *this* practice today exactly as you desire.

After my practice, I am thinking about:
My mind, breath, and Spirit feel:

Introspection: What did today's practice, curated by you, bring you? How will you maintain consistency in your practice beyond the confines of this 21-day guide? What brought you this far? What could keep you pursuing this practice and its many gifts?

Forging Ahead

Of course, circle back at any time and expand on your thoughts. Relearning and unlearning are necessary steps in the path. Return to these pages and their content whenever you feel inclined to check back in with the foundations of Nidra, and reconnect to the space you were resting in upon your first read. As you proceed beyond these pages, may your cyclical ways carry you through and along your varied journeys. May Nidra remain with you for as long as it is of benefit. May your path unfurl with increasing clarity, potent awareness, and joyous learning all the while.

Nidra Yoga for Beginners

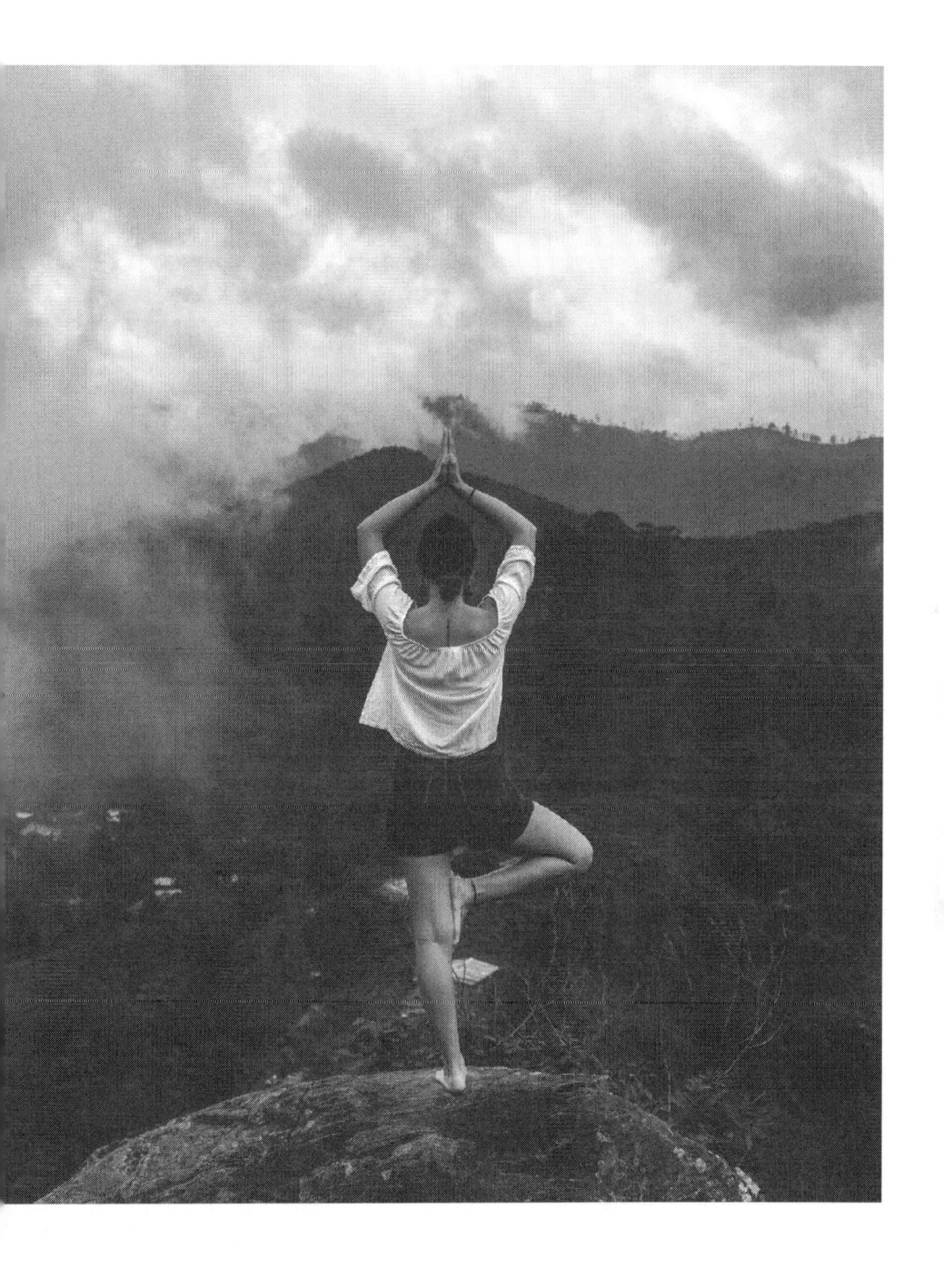

Reviews

Reviews and feedback help improve this book and the author. If you enjoy this book, we would greatly appreciate it if you could take a few moments to share your opinion and post a review on Amazon.

© 2019

Printed in Poland
by Amazon Fulfillment
Poland Sp. z o.o., Wrocław